D1132296

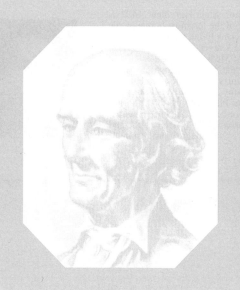

The author, Alain Horvilleur, M.D. is one of the foremost homeopathic physicians living today. A graduate of the University of Lyon (France) School of Medicine, he is President of the International Homeopathic Medical Organization and teaches Homeopathy at the University of Lyon School of Pharmacy. He is the author of a number of books on Homeopathy, both for the general public and for medical professionals.

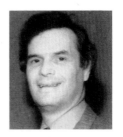

The author would like to express gratitude to JulianWinston for his invaluable help and would like to thank Jack Moseley for his kind assistance in editing this book.

Alain Horvilleur, M.D.

President
of the International Homeopathic Medical Organization

The Family Guide to Homeopathy

Translated by D. Clausen,
English version revised by the author.

General warning:

The conditions for which self-treatment is appropriate usually fall into the following categories:

1) They are self-limiting; that is, they will resolve themselves in time without intervention.

2) They do not require the immediate care of a physician.

3) They do not require complex medical diagnosis or monitoring.

In any case, consult your physician if condition worsens or persists.

The Family Guide to Homeopathy is not intended to replace the medical advice of the reader's own physician or to contradict the medical or surgical treatment decisions of any ailment of the reader by a licensed physician. In no way is the information in this book to be considered as a prescription of treatment of medicine for any disease without the knowledge and consent of a physician personally familiar with the reader's health background. Consult a physician in person whenever more information is required about any ailment or health topic.

Neither the author, the copyright holder, nor the publisher authorizes the use of their names or any material in this book for the endorsement, sale or advertisement of any medical, paramedical, or healthcare related product, publication, apparatus.

No material from this book may be used, quoted, or reproduced without the permission of the author, copyright holder or publisher.

*
* *

The Family Guide to Homeopathy is read in a number of English speaking countries. For the sake of completeness, most of the homeopathic medicines applicable to the ailments indexed in this book are discussed although not all of these medicines may be available in your country.

Homeopathy is a therapeutic method which clinically applies the Law of Similars and uses medically active substances at weak or infinitesimal doses.

■ **A WORD ABOUT USING THIS BOOK**

By Dr. Alain Horvilleur, the author.

The Family Guide to Homeopathy is a useful, practical book of information about the field of medicine known as **Homeopathy.** This guidebook is designed to introduce the non-physician reader to the general principles of Homeopathy and to help him choose and take homeopathic medicines in the safest and most effective way.

Over 1,000 different topics covering the range of common ailments are discussed so that a well-informed choice may be made about which problems might best be treated by Homeopathy and which cannot. *The Guide* is conveniently arranged in alphabetical order, like a dictionary, so that you and your family may refer to it quickly and easily to find the information you are looking for at any given time. A correct understanding of your health problems and of Homeopathy will allow the proper selection of treatment. Sometimes this selection can be made on your own, sometimes a doctor trained in homeopathic medicine should help you with it. This is an important point to keep in mind, and *The Guide* is intended to make the distinction clear when appropriate.

■ DEFINITION OF HOMEOPATHY

Homeopathy is a therapeutic method which clinically applies the **Law of Similars** and uses medically active substances at weak or **infinitesimal doses.**

The Law of Similars

The fundamental principle of Homeopathy is the LAW OF SIMILARS. This law formulates the parallel action or similarity between the toxic potential of a substance and its therapeutic action.

For those wishing to apply homeopathic therapeutics, this law necessarily implies knowing the action of different substances in healthy persons.

For example:

Bee venom causes pinkish-red swelling in healthy individuals. The symptoms appear suddenly with an itching and burning sensation and are relieved by applications of cold water. *In infinitesimal doses, the same venom improves or cures* itchy, burning eruptions of sudden onset which are relieved by cold compresses. However, this type of eruption has a different origin, which may be sunburn, or urticaria due to a hypersensitivity to foods or drugs.

Homeopathy is based on a 1st premise:

Any biologically active substance can cause a set of symptoms to appear in a healthy person; these symptoms are *characteristic of the substance* used.

A 2nd premise:

Anyone suffering from a particular disease shows a set of symptoms which is *characteristic of the disease.* These pathological symptoms can be defined as being "changes in the way the person feels or behaves."

A 3rd premise:

The cure, which is confirmed by the objective disappearance of pathological symptoms, may be obtained by taking the substance whose experimental symptoms in healthy persons are most similar to the patient's own symptoms, provided this substance has been prepared homeopathically.

Homeopathy is a method of *individualized therapy.*

Homeopathic treatment involves *individual* symptoms, and homeopathic remedies act as *specific* stimulants to assist the body's defenses, as opposed to traditional remedies which act coercively.

Homeopathic medicines act in the same way as our system's defense reactions. They stimulate the natural defenses of the body in order to make them more effective and, thus, work with the body rather than against it.

This is the reason why, in Homeopathy, only infinitesimal doses are needed: an overly strong dose could aggravate the patient's condition.

The Infinitesimal Dose

In order to spare the patient unpleasant reactions due to a worsening of his or her condition, stimulation must not be too strong. It must act as a support or an encouragement to the organism.

It was after years of experimenting that Samuel Hahnemann, founder of the homeopathic method, came to the following conclusion: *"In order to bring about prompt, gentle, and lasting improvement, you most often need to use infinitesimal doses."* And, because these doses are infinitesimal or extremely weak, they are considered safe.

Hahnemann himself codified the preparation methods of these doses, which have changed little over the years:

Homeopathic medicines are made by successive steps of diluting or attenuating a starting or base substance into a weaker or *infinitesimal dose.* These doses are dynamized in dilutions called *Homeopathic potencies.* A medium potency of 7 or 9 C is usually recommended for general symptom levels. (C stands for Hahnemannian Centesimal, which means a 1/100th dilution. A 7 C preparation has been diluted to the 1/100th seven successive times; a 9 C preparation diluted to the 1/100th nine successive times, etc...). Each deconcentration undergoes shaking in a laboratory instrument called a *potentizer* (or dynamizer).

Homeopathic medicines come in three principal forms: *pellets* (granules #20 and globules #35), *drops,* and *tablets.* Granules #20 are packaged in unit-dose tubes and the entire contents of a tube is to be taken at once; globules #35 are packaged in multi-dose tubes and are generally taken three at a time. For convenience sake, globules #35 are called "pellets" throughout *The Guide.*

Both sizes of pellets are taken by mouth, and the best route of absorption to achieve their maximum effect is *under the tongue.* Whatever homeopathic medicine or medicines are taken, the dose is the same for all ages—children as well as adults. Once a remedy has relieved your symptoms you may stop taking it. You will find a detailed explanation of the pharmaceutical preparation of homeopathic medicines and how to take them properly (what to do and what not to do) under the heading, **Homeopathic medicines.** It's an important part of this dictionary and should not be overlooked.

■ Looking Up A Topic About Your Health

Most of the common health problems that affect people are discussed in *The Guide.* You will usually find the answer about an illness or its treatment by looking under its heading in the text. For example, under **Migraines,** you'll find a description of this particular type of headache and a homeopathic medicine best suited to each type of migraine headache according to its associated symptoms.

For some health problems, more than one kind of homeopathic medicine may be recommended since one treatment might work better for some people than for others. Also, in some cases, more than one treatment works best. Homeopathy is always an individualized therapy, and the non-toxicity of homeopathic preparations affords you the choice and safety, should you hesitate between several, of taking more than one recommended homeopathic medicine at the same time.

If a homeopathic treatment does not seem to work, you should consult a doctor trained in homeopathic medicine. He or she may be able to help you find a treatment that's more adapted to your individual needs.

Sometimes you may want to look up a topic out of sheer curiosity. *The Guide* is also a good manual for answering many of the questions that you or your family may have about staying in good health and preventing some health problems before they occur.

■ Looking Up A Homeopathic Medication

Most of the 200 homeopathic medicines commonly in use are discussed in *The Guide*. You will find them listed alphabetically, like all the topics. Under the name of each medication, there is information about the base substance of the medicine, the type of symptoms for which it is suited, and clinical indications for its use.

The Family Guide to Homeopathy has been written to help you and your family understand the positive role that Homeopathy can play in your everyday healthcare. It can be an invaluable guide in helping you select your own homeopathic remedies, but it will also indicate when—and why—you need to seek the advice of a doctor. In some cases, a physician trained in the discipline of Homeopathy should be consulted before you take any medication. *The Guide* will make it clear when you need to seek professional medical advice and when a particular disease or health problem is not within the realm of Homeopathy.

For most of the common health concerns and health problems of families, Homeopathy provides an excellent and natural way of taking care of ourselves and our loved ones. As you will see by using this book, Homeopathy is more than just a therapy, it is a way of thinking that brings us closer to nature—our own nature.

A

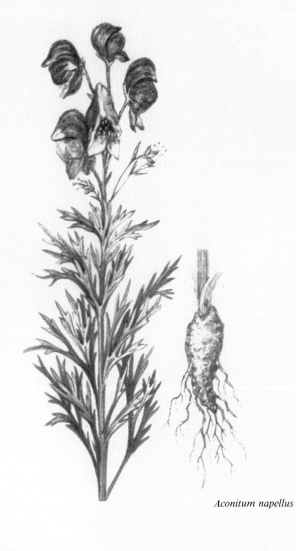

Aconitum napellus

Abdomen

▷ *See* **Stomach.**

Abies canadensis

Base substance: Hemlock spruce.

Characteristic signs and symptoms:
Stomachache accompanied by
constant hunger; distension of the
stomach; a sensation of cold between
the shoulders.

Main clinical use: Atonia of the
stomach, gastritis.

Abies nigra

Base substance: Black spruce.

Characteristic signs and symptoms:
Sensation of "an egg stuck in the
stomach" accompanied by
stomachache following meals, and
occasional coughing.

Main clinical use: Poor digestion.

Abscess, boil (Furuncle)

WARNING: Consult your physician.

There is a difference between an
abscess (the collection of pus inside a
natural or artificially produced cavity)
and a boil (a particular kind of abscess
of a skin gland or hair follicle caused
by "staphylococcus" germs). The
homeopathic treatment will be the
same.

General treatment

Beginning of the abscess:
- If the skin is pinkish in color,
  APIS MELLIFICA 9 C,
  three pellets three times a day.
- If the skin is red,
  BELLADONNA 9 C,
  three pellets three times a day.

For a fully-formed abscess,
HEPAR SULPHURIS CALCAREUM 3 X,
two tablets three times a day.

For persistent abscesses,
SILICEA 9 C,
three pellets three times a day,
until the abscess disappears.

Topical treatment

Use CALENDULA ointment.

*WARNING: If condition persists,
discontinue use of the above remedies
and consult your physician.*

▷ *Also see* **Anthrax, Pharyngitis** (for
abscess of the throat), **Styes, Teeth**
(for dental abscess).

Abulia

This disease is essentially
characterized by loss or impairment of
willpower. The patient no longer
wishes to do anything nor does he or
she have the strength alone to
overcome his or her inactivity or
idleness. This condition is difficult to
treat because it requires not only
medical attention but also the patient's
active participation, which is often
hard to obtain.

Treatment:
Try AURUM METALLICUM 9 C, three
pellets three times a day (at least
several days).
In any case, a homeopathic physician
should be consulted.

Accidental asphyxiation
(Aftercare for)

Seek competent medical assistance.
Following professional treatment, take:
   CARBO VEGETABILIS 5 C,
   three pellets three times a week for
   three months.

Accidents

▷ *See* **Accidental asphyxiation,
Fractures, Injuries, Sprains.**

Acetone

*WARNING: If condition persists,
consult your physician.*
Acetone can be found in urine
(chemically identifiable) as well as in
exhaled air (causing the typical
"apple" breath odor) when the
patient's sugar reserves are
insufficient. Fat reserves are then
burned to make up for the lack of
sugar, and acetone is a by-product of
this degradation.

Treatment:
   SENNA 9 C,
   three pellets every hour until
   improvement.

Preventive treatment:
Consult a homeopathic physician who
will in most cases choose between:
   LYCOPODIUM CLAVATUM,
   PHOSPHORUS and SEPIA.

Acidity

Acidity in the digestive tract:
• The remedy to use in case of acid

vomiting, stomach acidity or acidic
stools is:
   IRIS VERSICOLOR 9 C,
   three pellets three times a day.

General acidity in perspiration:
• If a child's perspiration has an acid
odor:
   CALCAREA CARBONICA 9 C,
   three pellets three times a day.

Acne (Juvenile)

Juvenile acne is characterized by
blackheads (comedones), pimples or
purplish scars, or occasionally all
three. The skin merely acts as a setting
for this disease whose causes may be
of an infectious, circulatory, hormonal
or psychic nature. Prolonged treatment
using antibiotics should be considered
only in severe cases; although
antibiotics do a spectacular job of
clearing up the acne at the beginning,
relapses nearly always occur due to the
existence of non-microbian causes.
Generally speaking, the various topical
ointments available are relatively
ineffective for these same reasons.
Hi-dose antibiotic treatment also has
the disadvantage of destroying a large
part of the normal intestinal flora.
On the other hand, mechanical
treatments (abrasion, dry ice), when
applied by competent specialists, can
help to complete the homeopathic
treatment.

• For blackheads,
   SELENIUM 9 C,
   three pellets three times a day.
• For pimples,
   KALI BROMATUM 9 C,
   three pellets three times a day.
• For purplish scars,
   ANTIMONIUM TARTARICUM 9 C,
   three pellets three times a day.

Local treatment:
Use CALENDULA ointment.

▷ Patients having suffered from acne for a long time should consult a homeopathic physician who will devise a preventive treatment after examining the patient's general characteristics.

Acne rosacea

This disease is completely different from juvenile acne. It is frequently found in women in their forties. These patients suffer from circulatory disorders characterized by a dilation of blood vessels in the face, especially the cheeks, causing blotching.
Take:
SANGUINARIA CANADENSIS 9 C,
CARBO ANIMALIS 9 C,
alternate three pellets of each,
three times daily.
For persistent cases, consult a physician.

Aconitum napellus
(or Aconite)

Base substance: Aconite.

Suitable for:
The aftereffects of exposure to cold, and the aftereffects of fright in patients who are usually in good health.

Characteristic signs and symptoms:
Anxiety with fear of death; a red face; arterial congestion; a high temperature without perspiration; dry mucosa and skin; a hacking cough; violent palpitations; "pins and needle"-like pains; the sudden and brutal onset of all of these symptoms.

Main clinical uses:
The beginning of many infectious diseases; fever, dry skin, intense thirst, restlessness, all associated with colds

of sudden onset; laryngitis; facial neuralgia; acute fits of minor anxiety.

WARNING: If condition worsens or persists for more than 72 hours, check with your physician.

Acrocyanosis

In this disease, the limbs turn cold, blue and sweaty because of passive circulatory congestion. A doctor must always be consulted when this illness appears. Your doctor may recommend:
CARBO VEGETABILIS 9 C,
LACHESIS 9 C,
PULSATILLA 9 C,
alternate three pellets of each,
three times a day.

Acupuncture and Homeopathy

Acupuncture and Homeopathy complement each other, and many physicians may choose to apply them simultaneously. Each of these methods stimulates the organism's natural system of defense, either by using needles or by using a remedy chosen according to the Law of Similars (see **Homeopathic theory**). Acupuncture and Homeopathy are both **natural** forms of medicine. They are non-toxic, and their effectiveness is comparable and complementary.

May the two methods be used together?

They are perfectly compatible. Acupuncture often has an immediate effect while Homeopathy, at least in long-term illnesses, acts after several

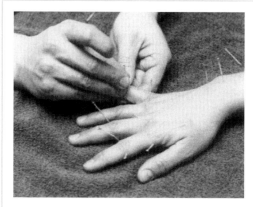

Acupuncture is one of the oldest forms of medicine in the world. The first book based on this theory dates back to 2,500 B.C.

weeks or months of treatment. It may be beneficial to begin both therapeutic treatments at the same time. Sometimes, however, the physician may prefer to use only one of the two treatments to judge its effectiveness for the case in question.

Addison's disease

This is an organic disease of the adrenal glands that causes the glands to produce an insufficient quantity of hormones.
It cannot be treated by Homeopathy.

Adenitis, Adenopathy

▷ *See* **Lymph nodes.**

Adenoids

Hypertrophy of the lymphoid nodules at the back of the throat or nasopharynx is one sign of recurrent throat and nasal inflammation (see **Rhinopharyngitis**) and may be complicated by otitis.
Homeopaths consider the adenoids to be a defense system against infection that should be left in place: removing them surgically gives germs the chance to travel further into the respiratory system. A long-term homeopathic treatment established by a homeopathic physician will help to avoid rhinopharyngitis and otitis without recourse to an operation.

Adenoma of the prostate gland

▷ *See* **Prostate gland disorders.**

Adynamia

▷ *See* **Fatigue** (fortifiers).

Aesculus hippocastanum

Base substance: Horse chestnut.

Suitable for: Venous congestion associated with a sedentary lifestyle.

Characteristic signs and symptoms: Purplish hemorrhoids with a sensation of rectal fullness or "pins and needles," and minimal bleeding; dryness of the rectal mucosa; varicose veins; shooting pains in the lumbar region.

Main clinical uses: Hemorrhoids, lumbago, varicose veins.

Aesculus hippocastanum

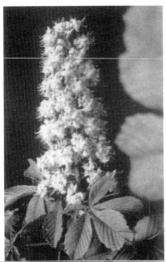

Aethusa cynapium

Base substance: Lesser or Garden hemlock.

Suitable for: Small, emaciated infants with pronounced facial features.

Characteristic signs and symptoms: Intolerance to milk by babies (the milk is brought up as soon as it has been swallowed), accompanied by watery diarrhea and prostration, sometimes convulsions; decreased attention span.

WARNING: It should be stressed that convulsions in infants are a medical emergency requiring examination by a doctor.

Main clinical uses: Gastroenteritis; reviewing for school exams.

Agalactia

Insufficient milk supply in the breasts.

▷ *See* **Breast-feeding.**

Agaricus muscarius

Base substance: Bug or fly agaric.

Characteristic signs and symptoms: Chilblains (frostbite) of the hands and feet with redness, burning, icy-prickling sensation, or itching; muscle spasms; a lack of coordination of movements.

Main clinical uses: Circulatory disorders: *WARNING - This disease is serious. Contact your physician immediately for treatment recommendation.* Chilblains; hangover symptoms; nervous tics.

Agoraphobia

It's often mistakenly thought that agoraphobia is a fear of crowds. Actually, it is the dread of being in or crossing open spaces: for example, a public square with no one in it. The sufferer prefers to sneak along, pressed against the walls rather than walking straight across it. The term "agoraphobia" stems from the Greek word "agora" meaning "public square," and "phobia" meaning "fear." Take ARGENTUM NITRICUM 9 C, either three pellets three times a day for a few months if the condition is severe, or simply three pellets before leaving home.

Agraphis nutans

Base substance: Wild hyacinth.

Characteristic signs and symptoms: Inflammation and hypertrophy of the adenoids; inflammation of the throat extending to the ears.

Main clinical uses: Temporary hearing impairment caused by pharyngeal disorders; inflammation of the adenoids with complications affecting the ears: *WARNING* - *These diseases are serious. Contact your physician immediately for treatment recommendation.*

Air sickness

▷ *See* **Travel sickness.**

Air swallowing

▷ *See* **Eructation.**

Albuminuria

▷ *See* **Urine test.**

Alcoholism

Alcoholism is a serious social problem that has, in many cases, been treated successfully by Homeopathy.
In the last century, a Frenchman Dr. Gallavardin wrote a book, *The Treatment of Alcoholism by Homeopathy.* This book is still published and available in the United States. It remains, to this day, a valuable resource.

Aletris farinosa

Base substance: Star grass.

Suitable for: Women bothered by fatigue, anemia, or gynecological problems.

Characteristic signs and symptoms: Extreme fatigue; lack of appetite; a heavy feeling in the uterus; excessive menstruation ("heavy periods"); tendency to prolapsed female organs.

Main clinical use: Women with a prolapsed uterus who experience fatigue.

Allergy

Some patients successfully undergo a "desensitization" treatment to the substance responsible for their allergy. Because these people don't generally consult a homeopathic physician, it's difficult to know what proportion of true successes are obtained by desensitization treatment. However, the failure rate is probably high since the homeopathic doctor sees many patients come to him or her after having subjected themselves to years of weekly injections of various "allergens" in a vain attempt to be cured of their allergies.

The treatment of allergies by Homeopathy often succeeds in those cases where everything else has failed. Admittedly it is a long-term treatment, as the product responsible for the allergy cannot always be eliminated from the patient's surroundings, but it's an easy treatment to take.

Allergy tests may sometimes be of help to the homeopathic physician. Besides the usual allergies to household dust and feathers (almost predictable for most allergy sufferers), it would be helpful to find out if the patient is allergic to pet fur, a germ, or a commercial household product. If so, the cause can sometimes be eliminated before deciding on a treatment.

All types of allergies may be treated with Homeopathy: **urticaria (hives), eczema, asthma,** allergic **colds** and **hay fever** (see these entries). *The Guide* can suggest several helpful treatments for temporary bouts. If you have suffered from a particular allergy for quite some time, however, you should consult a homeopathic physician for an in-depth treatment. (Allergy is one of the most typical examples of the idea of "terrain"—see this entry).

Allium cepa

Base substance: the Common onion.

Characteristic signs and symptoms: Nasal inflammation with discharge irritating the upper lip; inflammation of the eyes with, on the contrary, a non-irritating discharge; harsh bouts of sneezing; painful vocal cords, especially when coughing; an unpleasant tickling feeling in the ears when suffering from a cold, improved by the open air.

Main clinical uses: Common cold, hay fever.

Allopathy

What is Allopathy?

Allopathy is the medicine of "opposites"—that is, "the medicine different from the disease." (Etymologically, from the Greek words "allos" (other) and "pathos" (disease)). This type of medicine is the most widespread form of therapy practiced by general practitioners today.

Allopathy is founded on the principle that the remedy prescribed by the doctor should act against the patient's symptoms, which is why **anti**biotics, **anti**coagulants, **anti**depressants, etc. are used in Allopathy. Homeopathy takes the opposite approach; it advocates using medicines that are prescribed in accordance with the **Law of Similars** (see **Homeopathic theory**).

Why do allopathic doctors seldom recommend that their patients consult a homeopathic physician?

They could easily make the recommendation in cases where their own types of medicine fail to work. But the vast majority of allopathic physicians know nothing about Homeopathy.

Not a single course about Homeopathy is even offered to students in most medical schools. General practitioners cannot develop the reflex to send their patients to see a homeopathic specialist without having been "taught" to do so. Hopefully, the present attitude will evolve. After all, the future of medicine belongs to a team approach among health professionals.

What should you do if you're already taking an allopathic treatment when you consult a homeopathic physician?

The homeopath should decide what is best. If he feels it's possible, he may stop the allopathic treatment, replacing it with a homeopathic one. Sometimes he may see fit to use both treatments at the same time. For example, it would be indispensable for a patient with heart disease who is already taking anticoagulants and cardiotonic drugs to continue, but nothing says that he or she can't take a homeopathic treatment for a liver condition at the same time.

Consider the case of a depressed patient who manages to "survive" thanks to an allopathic tranquilizer. When consulting a homeopathic physician for the first time, it is recommended that the patient "gently" change over from that form of therapy to a homeopathic one.

At first, both the allopathic and the homeopathic treatments are administered together under competent medical supervision. Gradually, the allopathic medication is spaced further and further apart as progress allows, sparing the patient the uneasy feeling of "missing" his earlier medication.

The allopathic tranquilizer may still be held in reserve in case it is really needed from time to time. The main treatment is therefore a homeopathic one, but some patients feel the need to calm their anxiety with tranquilizers for a day or two during a difficult

moment; there's no reason to deny them this. The same goes for migraine headaches: the long-term homeopathic treatment is best, but an allopathic medication may relieve some acute pain until the homeopathic treatment has had time to work.

Although the term "Allopathy," coined by Hahnemann (see **History of Homeopathy**), may be known by the general public, the homeopathic physician still encounters people who do not know how to refer to Allopathy except as "the other type of medicine." In fact, one type of medicine, Allopathy, is not "chemical"-based, and the other type, Homeopathy, "plant"-based:

- Homeopathy also uses medicines derived from the mineral kingdom; they could, consequently, be termed "chemicals" in the broad sense of the term. Examples are: PHOSPHORICUM ACIDUM (phosphoric acid) and SULPHUR IODATUM (sulfur iodide).

- Allopathy, like Homeopathy, also uses plants. Digitalis (foxglove), for example, and its alkaloid, digitaline, are very effective in certain cases of heart failure. Doctors use these medicines in accordance with very precise prescription rules. Just because they're derived from plants does not mean that they should not be handled with precaution.

It's important not to oversimplify matters by thinking that "chemical medicine is dangerous and plant-based medicine is mild in its action."

Aloe socotrina

Base substance: Aloes.

Suitable for: Sedentary patients.

Characteristic signs and symptoms: Burning diarrhea with large amounts of mucus; a feeling of fullness in the abdomen; poor anal sphincter control with occasional external prolapse of rectal mucosa; hemorrhoids during bouts of diarrhea.

Main clinical uses: Diarrhea; hemorrhoids; inflammation of the rectum.

Alopecia

Baldness, loss of hair.

▷ *See* **Hair.**

Altitude sickness

Some people suffer symptoms of their ailments from being in a mountainous or high altitude region. The best way to avoid this is simply not to go there! However, if you have to spend some time in the mountains, take three pellets of the following remedy three times a day:

ARGENTUM NITRICUM 9 C,
for dizziness or the sensation that the mountains are closing in on you.

Don't overtax yourself in the mountains. Slow down, and see a doctor if you don't feel better soon.

Alumina

Base substance: Aluminum oxide.
Characteristic signs and symptoms: Dryness of the skin and mucous membranes; various types of paralysis; constipation due to paralysis of the rectum and dryness of the mucosa—the patient must make an enormous effort to pass a bowel movement; anal itching; abundant

white vaginal discharge (leukorrhea); symptoms are aggravated by eating potatoes.

Main clinical uses: Constipation; white vaginal discharge.

Amenorrhea

Absence of menstruation.

▷ *See* **Menstrual periods.**

Anacardium orientale

Base substance: Marking nut.
Suitable for: The consequences of nervous strain.

Characteristic signs and symptoms: Sudden loss of memory; sensation of contradictory will; incapacity to make the slightest mental effort; irritability; a feeling of emptiness in the pit of the stomach; symptoms are relieved when the patient eats.

Main clinical uses:
Mental and emotional disorders.
Loss of memory: *WARNING — This disease is serious. You should consult your physician for advice.*

Analogy

In some homeopathic books, the authors speak of the "Law of Analogy" instead of the "Law of Similars" (see **Homeopathic theory**) when referring to the basic fundamentals of Homeopathy. In this restricted sense, the two terms have the same meaning. It would be preferable, however, to reserve the term "analogy" for the following definition, which is wider and more generally accepted: "a similarity drawn by the imagination between two or more essentially different subjects of thought." Analogy can be seen everywhere. It may exist between two objects in so far as their shape, color, use, etc. For example, there is an analogy between your own heart and your car's engine: both function rhythmically, both run on an indispensable liquid, and both play a very important role in the complex organism which they are a part of. Both can even be replaced with spare parts! There does exist an analogy between them, but the similarity stops there; they are by no means identical.

The Law of Similars is a particular kind of analogy. There are points in common between the clinical appearance of healthy individuals who experimentally ingest a given substance, and sick patients who exhibit the same symptoms due to their illness. There is indeed an analogy, but it's more than merely "similarity established by the imagination." *It is a rational approach to the question.*

Anemia

The causes of anemia are many, and some of them require immediate medical attention. You should, therefore, always check with your doctor if you suspect you're anemic. The homeopathic doctor will often use both Allopathy and Homeopathy in his treatment plan. Allopathy will provide what is low or lacking in the organism (iron, vitamin B_{12}), while Homeopathy will supply the "catalysts" needed to make the allopathic treatment more effective. Figuratively speaking, merely having

the right amount of coal for the job is not enough; one needs a good fan or bellows to bring the coal to red hot. While waiting to see your doctor or in minor cases of anemia, you may take the following medicines:

- For anemia with fatigue,
  CINCHONA OFFICINALIS 9 C,
  three pellets three times a day.
- For anemia with hot flashes,
  FERRUM METALLICUM 9 C,
  three pellets three times a day.
- For anemia with weight loss,
  NATRUM MURIATICUM 9 C,
  three pellets three times a day.

Anger

For pains secondary to anger:
COLOCYNTHIS 9 C,
three pellets every hour until pains have stopped.

For irritable adults:
NUX VOMICA 9 C,
three pellets three times a day.

For a restless, irritable child:
CHAMOMILLA 9 C,
three pellets three times a day.

▷ *See* **Character.**

Angioma

A red or purplish spot caused by the agglomeration of blood vessels on the skin. An angioma is congenital in origin and is also called a vascular nevus or "port wine stain."

If the angioma is small in size, give the child:
CALCAREA CARBONICA 9 C,
three pellets three times a day, ten days a month until symptoms disappear.

Animal bites

WARNING: Seek professional medical treatment immediately, then take:
    LACHESIS 5 C,
    LEDUM PALUSTRE 5 C,
    alternate three pellets of each,
    every hour.

Local treatment:
Apply CALENDULA ointment topically to minor wounds.

▷ *See* **Snake bites.**

Animals

Bites: ▷ *see* above entry.
Can animals be treated with Homeopathy? ▷ *see* **Homeopathic veterinarians.**
Fear of animals: ▷ *see* **Fear.**

Ankles

Pains in: ▷ *see* **Rheumatism.**
Sprains: ▷ *see* this entry.

Ankylosing spondylarthritis

Inflammatory rheumatism, particularly affecting the sacroiliac joint and the lower vertebrae. Only the early stages of this disease can be treated homeopathically. A medical consultation is warranted but you may take the following in the meantime:
    TUBERCULINUM NOSODE 12 C,
    three unit-dose tubes a week.

Annoyance
(Consequences of)

▷ *See* **Emotion.**

Anorexia

The medical term for lack of appetite (see **Appetite**).

▷ For cases of *anorexia nervosa* (an extreme aversion to food usually occurring in young women who lose a tremendous amount of weight and no longer have normal menstrual periods), it is absolutely necessary to consult a doctor. In the meantime, try giving:
    PULSATILLA 9 C,
    three pellets three times a day.

Anosmia

Loss of the sense of smell.

▷ *See* **Nose, Smell.**

Anthracinum

Base substance: Liver lysate of anthrax-infected rabbits.

Suitable for:
Infected or infection-prone cuts from an unclean instrument.

Characteristic signs and symptoms:
Spreading infection bordering on gangrene; burning pains; infiltration of the entire infected region.

Main clinical uses:
Anthrax, gangrene, septicemia, serious boils: *WARNING—These diseases are serious. Contact your physician immediately for treatment recommendation.*

Anthrax

WARNING: For this disease, you must consult your physician.

This is a purulent build-up under the skin from anthrax bacteria in wounds or abrasions, which may be accompanied by infiltration of surrounding tissue. Your doctor may recommend that you take:

ANTHRACINUM 9 C,
ARSENICUM ALBUM 9 C,
LACHESIS 9 C,
alternate three pellets of each, every hour.

WARNING: Discontinue use of the above remedies and check directly with your doctor if this treatment doesn't work rapidly; anthrax can spread to internal organs.

Antibiotics

Are antibiotics used in Homeopathy?

The homeopathic doctor is often asked this question by patients. Strictly speaking, there are no antibiotics used in Homeopathy: homeopathic medicines are not **specific** (see this entry) to a particular disease or infectious agent. When homeopathic medicines are judiciously chosen according to the symptoms of each individual case, they can be just as effective as antibiotics. A homeopathic physician who is thoroughly familiar with his *Materia Medica* (see this entry) can usually manage without antibiotics nine out of ten times at no undue risk to the patient. Homeopathic medicines act by stimulating the organism's natural defense mechanisms which, in turn, neutralize the microbe. The homeopathic remedy itself does not kill the germ like antibiotics do.

Can you take antibiotics while undergoing a long-term homeopathic treatment?

If at all possible, try using a correctly chosen homeopathic remedy before using antibiotics. Your homeopathic physician will help you choose.
If you consult an allopathic physician and he or she prescribes antibiotics for a short period, you may stop the homeopathic treatment temporarily. For longer periods, inform the homeopath who prescribed your long-term treatment.

Anticipation

▷ *See* **Anxiety.**

Antidotes and Neutralizers to Avoid

The following substances should be avoided as much as possible while taking a homeopathic treatment:
Camphor, chamomile and mint—which are generally considered to neutralize or counteract the action of homeopathic medicines.

This effect is certain with camphor. So, when using nose drops, always check the ingredients. The same goes for certain ointments that contain camphor (particularly counterirritants—liniments).

The neutralizing effect is less clear (although it is traditionally accepted as existing) with chamomile and mint.
If you choose to eat, drink or brush your teeth with something containing mint, it is advisable to do so at least two hours before or after taking your homeopathic medicine.

Antimonium crudum

Base substance: Black antimony sulfide.

Suitable for:
The aftereffects of bathing in cold water; indigestion; overeating; the aftereffects of drinking poor quality, acidy wine.

Characteristic signs and symptoms:
Coated tongue from overeating, as if it were covered by the skin of boiled milk; diarrhea with semi-solid, semi-liquid stools; hemorrhoids with secretion of much mucus; warts; thick, brittle nails.

Main clinical uses:
Diarrhea; gastric disorders; hemorrhoids; horny eczema; nail problems; warts.

WARNING: If condition worsens or persists for more than 72 hours, check with your physician.

Antimonium tartaricum
(or Tartarus emeticus)

Base substance: Double tartrate of antimony and potassium.

Suitable for:
The second stage of acute pulmonary diseases when the lung isn't able to eliminate whatever is congesting it.

Characteristic signs and symptoms:
Bronchial congestion with a great deal of mucus and loud respiratory noises; difficulty in spitting; sensation of asphyxiation; congested face, cold sweating; nausea, sleepiness; pustular eruptions.

Main clinical uses:
Cough usually accompanied by shortness of breath with difficulty in removal of mucus (the person is usually pale and tired); bronchitis; asthma; pneumonia; emphysema; the constitutional symptoms of chickenpox.

WARNING: If condition worsens or persists for more than 72 hours, check with your physician.

Anuria (Anuresis)

The absence of the act of urination or suppression of urine formation. Check with your physician but in the meantime, take:
APIS MELLIFICA 5 C,
CANTHARIS 5 C,
alternate three pellets of each, every fifteen minutes.

WARNING: If condition worsens or persists for more than 72 hours, check with your physician.

Anus

For mild disorders, the following medicines may be taken:

Anal incontinence:
ALOE SOCOTRINA 5 C,
three pellets three times a day.

Bleeding:
HAMAMELIS VIRGINICA 6 X,
10 drops three times during the day.

WARNING: If symptoms or bleeding persist, a physician must be consulted immediately because the bleeding considered by the individual may not be from the suspected rectal area.

Eczema:
GRAPHITES 9 C,
three pellets three times a day.

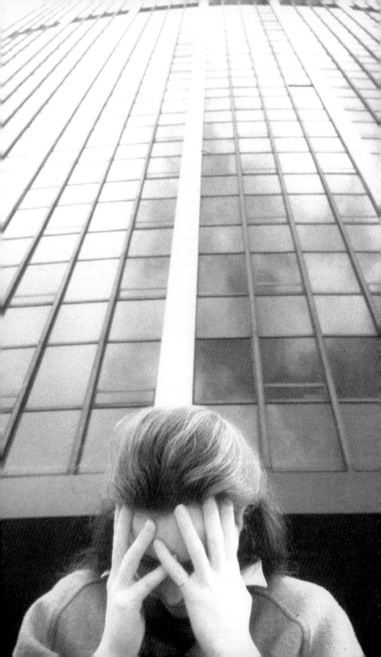

Fissures or cracking:
 GRAPHITES 9 C,
 NITRICUM ACIDUM 9 C,
 RATANHIA 9 C,
 alternate three pellets of each,
 three times a day.
Apply RATANHIA ointment locally,
once or twice a day.

Fistula:
Avoid having anal fistulas operated
on; this may cause relapses or even
bring on another illness. Always check
with a homeopathic physician. You
may take the following while waiting:
 BERBERIS VULGARIS 9 C,
 three pellets three times a day.

Hemorrhoids:
 ▷ *see* this entry.

Itching (pruritus):
● For no apparent reason,
 TEUCRIUM MARUM VERUM 9 C,
 three pellets three times a day.
● Due to worms,
 CINCHONA OFFICINALIS 9 C,
 three pellets three times a day.

Pain:
● Pain in the anus associated with
diarrhea,
 ALOE SOCOTRINA 9 C,
 three pellets three times a day.
● Pain in the anus while sitting,
 SEPIA 9 C,
 three pellets three times a day.
● Pain in the anus while walking,
 IGNATIA AMARA 9 C,
 three pellets three times a day.

Redness:
 SULPHUR 9 C,
 three pellets three times a day.

Anxiety

Anxiety is a feeling of worry (and
sometimes panic) which is
accompanied by physical symptoms:
palpitations, pain, sensation of
suffocation or contraction in the chest,
a "lump in the throat," etc.
If the symptoms are not physical but
psychological ones, we generally speak
of worry rather than anxiety.
Whatever the condition, take three
pellets of one of the following
medicines at the onset of attacks and
repeat every hour thereafter:

Depending on the cause:
● The dread of a future event
("anticipatory anxiety"),
 ARGENTUM NITRICUM 9 C.
● Bouts of anxiety during fever (with
fear of dying),
 ACONITUM NAPELLUS 9 C.
● The aftereffects of fright,
 ACONITUM NAPELLUS 9 C.
● A letdown or sad event,
 IGNATIA AMARA 9 C.
● Hot weather,
 PULSATILLA 9 C.

Depending on circumstances:
Worsening of anxiety:
● When one is alone,
 ARSENICUM ALBUM 9 C.
● At night,
 ARSENICUM ALBUM 9 C.
● Going down stairs,
 BORAX 9 C.
● At nightfall,
 PHOSPHORUS 9 C.

Anxiety is relieved:
● When eating,
 ANACARDIUM ORIENTALE 9 C.
● In the company of others,
 PHOSPHORUS 9 C.

Depending on sensations:
● A sensation of imminent death,
 ACONITUM NAPELLUS 9 C.
● Guilt complex,
 AURUM METALLICUM 9 C.
● Heavy feeling in the chest, or lump
in the throat,
 IGNATIA AMARA 9 C.
● An anxious feeling in the stomach,
 KALI CARBONICUM 9 C.
● A sensation of an imminent fainting
or weakness spell,
 MOSCHUS 9 C.

Anxiety can often be treated by Homeopathy.

Or depending on the consequences of anxiety:

• Mild palpitations,
ACONITUM NAPELLUS 9 C.
• Twitching,
AGARICUS MUSCARIUS 9 C.
• Claustrophobia, loss of balance while walking, irritation of the throat, hurriedness (trying to get everything over with), fear of heights,
ARGENTUM NITRICUM 9 C.
• Constant restlessness,
ARSENICUM ALBUM 9 C.
• Trembling,
GELSEMIUM SEMPERVIRENS 9 C.
• Stuttering,
STRAMONIUM 9 C.
• Cold sweats,
VERATRUM ALBUM 9 C.

If anxiety attacks occur more or less regularly, you should consult a homeopathic physician. The long-term preventive treatment should make them less frequent or eliminate them altogether. The treatment will not, however, prevent a case of reactive anxiety to a major life event (reactive anxiety to a real threat or loss is unavoidable; it's also an individual protection from danger). A good homeopathic treatment will make you less vulnerable to the minor annoyances that make up our daily lives.

▷ *See* **Fear.**

Apathy

The absence of emotion, indifference.

When you are unable to act positively because of psychological fatigue, take:
PHOSPHORICUM ACIDUM 9 C,
three pellets three times a day.

▷ *Also see* **Abulia** and **Depression.**

Aphonia

Loss of the voice.

▷ *See* **Laryngitis.**

Aphtha (pl./aphthae)

▷ *See* **Mouth.**

Apis mellifica

Base substance: the Common bee.

Characteristic signs and symptoms: Pinkish swelling of the skin and mucous membranes with pricking pains made worse by touching but relieved by cold compresses; although the person is feverish, he or she is not thirsty.

Main clinical uses: Insect bites; sunburn and hives; irritated skin; swelling due to disorders of the nerves around blood vessels, called Quincke's edema; burns; early stages of boils; frostbite; hay fever; flu-like symptoms; minor ovaritis; inflammation of the mucous membranes; rheumatism.

WARNING: If condition worsens or persists for more than 72 hours, check with your physician.

Appendicitis

The main symptoms of appendicitis are: pains in the right, lower side of the abdomen just below the navel; nausea; coated tongue; abnormal constipation.
Even for an experienced doctor,

appendicitis may be very difficult to diagnose. He or she may hesitate between two options: operating—only to discover that it was not appendicitis after all, or not operating—and taking the risk of having the appendicitis develop into peritonitis.

In any case, if you are in doubt, seek professional medical care.

Appetite

Excess appetite:

▷ *see* **Bulimia, Slimming.**

Lack of appetite:
CINCHONA OFFICINALIS 3 X,
GENTIANA LUTEA 3 X,
alternate three pellets of each,
three times a day.

Apprehension

▷ *See* **Emotion.**

Argentum nitricum

Base substance: Silver nitrate.

Suitable for:
People prone to worry or dread over important coming events (they may even tremble with apprehension).

Characteristic signs and symptoms:
Excessive burping; inflammation or ulceration of the mucous membranes; stomach pains made worse by sweets; diarrhea from anticipation; pricking pains in the throat with a constant need to clear the throat; loss of balance when walking; trembling; vertigo; claustrophobia; various kinds of fears; worry caused by anticipation; a desire for company; a nervous fear of leaving home.

Main clinical uses:
Gastritis, hiatal hernia, stomach ulcers, laryngitis, pharyngitis, conjunctivitis, mild anxiety, apprehension: *WARNING— These diseases are serious. You must consult your physician.*

Arnica montana

Base substance: Arnica.

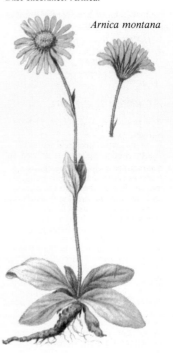

Arnica montana

Suitable for:
The consequences of various types of trauma and muscular strain.

Characteristic signs and symptoms:
Painful muscles; the bed feels hard because of muscular fatigue; condition is aggravated by the slightest touch; skin bruises of traumatic origin.

Main clinical uses:
Aftereffects of various types of trauma; sprains, painfully healing fractures, bruising, muscular aches, the prevention of post-surgical complications and the consequences of prolonged effort; training for sports.

WARNING: If condition worsens or persists for more than 72 hours, check with your physician.

Arsenicum album

Base substance: Arsenious anhydride.

Suitable for:
Food poisoning; people prone to be finicky, meticulous, always dressed up.

Characteristic signs and symptoms:
Nervous restlessness despite extreme fatigue; depressed patient often gives up hope of being cured and is afraid of dying; waking up around 1 a.m., feeling out of breath, particularly at night; thirst for small, frequently repeated quantities of cold water; foul-smelling diarrhea; burning pains relieved by warmth; dry skin with fine, powdery eczema like flour.

Main clinical uses:
Asthma; coryza; hay fever; various types of fever; any skin rash of sudden onset improved by heat; dry eczema; psoriasis; carbuncles; gastroduodenal ulcers; acute diarrhea resulting from spoiled food; minor depression; anxiety.

WARNING: If condition worsens or persists for more than 72 hours, check with your physician.

Artemisia abrotanum

Base substance: Southernwood.

Suitable for:
Irritable, thin children who sometimes look older than their real age.

Characteristic signs and symptoms:
Weight loss in infants, progressing from bottom to top of the body; alternating diarrhea and constipation; appetite (enormous) remains unaffected.

Main clinical use:
Digestive disorders in young infants, accompanied by weight loss:
WARNING—This disease is serious. Contact your physician immediately for treatment recommendation.

Arteriosclerosis
(Hardening of the Arteries)

A long-term homeopathic treatment is available to help prevent this disease from spreading and your homeopathic physician will work with you on establishing a treatment plan. Disorders, such as intermittent pain (mainly when walking), may be due to the obstruction of one or several arteries in the legs by narrowing and hardening of the arteries, especially with age. This condition can be complicated by spasms of the muscles around the arteries.

WARNING: Your doctor must be consulted immediately. A long-term treatment is essential.

Arthritis, arthrosis

▷ *See* **Rheumatism.**

Arum triphyllum

Base substance: Jack-in-the-pulpit.

Suitable for:
The consequences of voice strain (for singers, actors, public speakers).

Characteristic signs and symptoms:
Raw mucous membranes in which the patient has the intolerable feeling of "pins and needles"; excoriating nasal discharge; stopped-up nose; faltering, changing voice (hoarseness during a speech or while singing).

Main clinical uses:
Coryza; laryngitis.
Certain cases of scarlatina:
WARNING — This disease is serious. Contact your physician immediately for treatment recommendation.

Asafoetida

Base substance: Asafoetida

Characteristic signs and symptoms:
Spasms in the esophagus from the bottom upward creating a sensation of a rising lump in the throat; rancid belching; bone pains; skin ulcers.

Main clinical uses:
Inflammation of the bones; intestinal gas; varicose ulcers of the legs.

Ascites

An accumulation of liquid in the abdomen.
Homeopathy may help the classical treatment. Check with your doctor.

Asthenia

The medical term for weakness or fatigue.

▷ *See* **Fatigue.**

Asthma

WARNING: In all cases, consult a physician. If you are on prescription drugs, do not discontinue use except under your doctor's supervision.

How to treat an acute attack: see your physician immediately,
Then take three pellets of the following medicines every five minutes or every quarter hour according to the intensity of the attack:

Depending on the cause:
• Asthma at the end of an apparently cured episode of eczema,
    ARSENICUM ALBUM 9 C.
• Asthma caused by rainy weather,
    DULCAMARA 9 C.
• Asthma set off by being upset,
    IGNATIA AMARA 9 C.
• Asthma which comes on after meals,
    NUX VOMICA 9 C.

Depending on relieving or aggravating factors:
• Relief from asthma attacks by leaning forward,
    KALI CARBONICUM 9 C.
• Relief by kneeling and placing your head on the floor (Muslim prayer position),
    MEDORRHINUM 9 C.
• Relief by lying on your back with your arms spread apart,
    PSORINUM 9 C.
• Aggravation of asthma after sleeping,
    LACHESIS 9 C.

Depending on accompanying symptoms:
• Asthma with restlessness,
    ARSENICUM ALBUM 9 C.

• Asthma with a burning sensation in the chest,
ARSENICUM ALBUM 9 C.
• Asthma with much mucus in the chest, not coughed up so it causes loud snoring noises,
ANTIMONIUM TARTARICUM 9 C.
• Asthma with nausea,
IPECAC 9 C.
• Asthma with wheezing in the chest,
IPECAC 9 C.
• Asthma with small round gray bits of matter coughed up that look like tapioca,
KALI CARBONICUM 9 C.
• Asthma with pricking pains in the chest,
KALI CARBONICUM 9 C.
• Asthma with a sensation of warmth in the chest,
PHOSPHORUS 9 C.
If you hesitate between several of these medicines, alternate them every quarter of an hour. Homeopathy will not relieve every asthma attack. Allopathic medicines, particularly theophylline, will sometimes give better results.

Background treatment

The long-term preventive treatment of asthma lies well within the field of Homeopathy. The treatment will reduce frequency of attacks and ultimately help to eliminate them. Do not overly protect an asthmatic child—let him or her live as normal a life as other children. To make too much of an issue about your child's asthma might make it worse.

Atherosclerosis

A type of arteriosclerosis of the inner layer of artery walls caused by deposits of atheromatous, or lipid, plaques.

▷ *See* **Arteriosclerosis.**

Attention span (Short)

To be less forgetful or "absent-minded," take:
NATRUM MURIATICUM 9 C, three pellets three times a day, ten days a month over a period of several months.

Aurum metallicum

Base substance: Gold.

Suitable for:
Ruddy-faced, plethoric persons who are also melancholic; the aftereffects of emotional distress.

Characteristic signs and symptoms:
Sadness; despair; being "fed-up" with life; constant unhappiness with oneself; mood improved by music; tendency to irritability and anger; noise intolerance; palpitations; high blood pressure; congestion of the arteries; hot flashes; non-descended testicles.

Main clinical uses:
Depression.
High blood pressure:
WARNING— This disease is serious. Contact your physician immediately for treatment recommendation.

B

*"Homeopathy is the most advanced
and refined method of
treating patients economically and nonviolently."*
MAHATMA GANDHI

Baldness

Preventive measures are necessary.

▷ *See* **Hair.**

Baryta carbonica

Base substance: Barium carbonate.

Suitable for:
A child who is physically, mentally or emotionally delayed; an elderly person with a tendency to infantile behavior.

Characteristic signs and symptoms:
Infantile behavior; lack of memory; speech difficulties; large tonsils; sensitivity to cold; high blood pressure; sebaceous cysts of the scalp; foul-smelling, sweaty feet.

Main clinical uses:
Developmental delay in children; chronic tonsil infections; laryngitis; bronchitis; sebaceous cysts; memory loss.
High blood pressure: *WARNING - This disease is serious. You should consult your physician for advice.*

Bee Sting

▷ *See* **Insect bites.**

Bedsore (Decubitus ulcer)

Contact ulcerations of the skin, often crusted or weeping, that occur to bedridden, immobile patients from long contact with the bed. At the beginning, they may be treated by Homeopathy.

General treatment:
    ARNICA MONTANA 9 C,
    LACHESIS 9 C,
    alternate three pellets of each, three times a day.

Local treatment:
Mix equal amounts of
    ARNICA MONTANA M.T.,
    CALENDULA M.T.,
    (enough to make 1 fl.oz.)
Apply this mixture to the bedsores twice a day.

Bedwetting (in children)

▷ *See* **Enuresis.**

Belching

▷ *See* **Eructation.**

Belladonna

Base substance: Belladonna.

Suitable for:
Acute, infectious diseases accompanied by a high temperature, especially in children.

WARNING: Any sudden high fever, especially in infants and children, should be reported to your family doctor. Delirium or convulsions with fever are absolute medical emergencies and should be seen immediately by a doctor, or in an Emergency Room—don't wait to use Belladonna in this case, get to a doctor by phone or in person.

Characteristic signs and symptoms:
Sudden onset of the symptoms in a person who is usually in good health; high temperature, over 102° F, accompanied by intense thirst and a red, hot face and lips; dilated pupils; delirium caused by a fever or a state of minor depression; twitching; redness and dryness of the oral mucosa; throbbing pains; various types of swelling and eruptions. The person is sensitive to light, noise, and being moved.

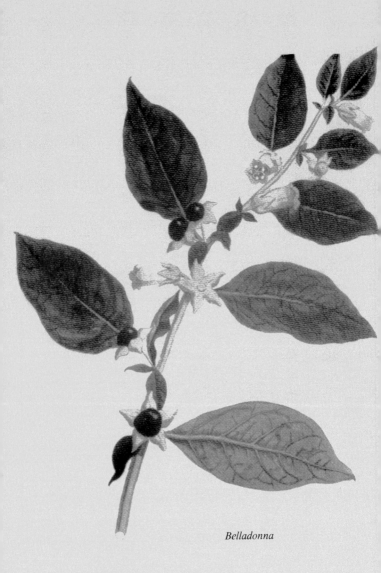

Belladonna

Main clinical uses:
Colds of sudden onset with sore throat, head congestion, fever, intense sweating; otitis; conjunctivitis; measles; scarlatina; skin burns; onset of an abscess; migraines; neuralgia; biliary cramps; kidney stones; gout.

WARNING: If condition worsens or persists for more than 72 hours, check with your physician.

Benzoicum acidum

Base substance: Benzoic acid.

Characteristic signs and symptoms:
Pain in the knees, especially due to gout; strong-smelling urine.

Main clinical use:
Gout and its accompanying urinary complications: *WARNING - This disease is serious. Contact your physician immediately for treatment recommendation.*

Berberis vulgaris

Base substance: Barberry

Characteristic signs and symptoms:
Pains radiating in all directions from their point of origin, particularly in the urinary tract, the liver, and the lumbar region; circular skin eruptions healing from the center outward with pigmented spots on the outer edge; anal fistula.

Main clinical uses:
Temporary relief from pain caused by gallstones or kidney stones; lumbago; acne; eczema; anal fistula. Rheumatism with urinary complications: *WARNING - This disease is serious. You should consult your physician for advice.*

Bile ducts

For pains in the bile ducts, take:
CHELIDONIUM MAJUS 9 C,
MAGNESIA PHOSPHORICA 9 C,
alternate three pellets of each, every hour or three times a day depending on the severity of the pain.

For hepatic colic, ▷ *see* **Colic.**

For infection of the bile duct or cholecystitis, check with a doctor.

For gallstones, ▷ *see* **Calculi.**

Birth control pill

▷ *See* **Contraception.**

Birthmarks

▷ *See* **Nevus.**

Blackheads

▷ *See* **Acne (Juvenile).**

Bladder (Irritation of the)

Cystitis: ▷ *see* **Urinary infection.**

Benign tumors, polyps: If removed too often they may grow back more quickly. Consult a homeopathic physician. He or she may provide you with a long-term treatment that reduces the need for surgical intervention. While waiting to see the doctor, take:
NITRICUM ACIDUM 5 C,
THUJA OCCIDENTALIS 5 C,
alternate three pellets three times a day.

Bleeding

Various types of bleeding are listed below as well as an immediate treatment suggestion for each. You should still check with your doctor if any of them occur.

Depending on how serious the bleeding is, take three pellets of one of the following remedies either every five minutes, every hour, or three times a day.

Anus:
COLLINSONIA CANADENSIS 5 C.

WARNING: If symptoms or bleeding persist, a physician must be consulted immediately because the bleeding discovered by the individual may not be from the suspected rectal area.

Nosebleeding (epistaxis):
Hypertension may be related to a spontaneous (untraumatic) nosebleed. You should be examined by a doctor. If bleeding is heavy, or if it lasts more than several minutes, take:
CINCHONA OFFICINALIS 5 C,
MILLEFOLIUM 4 C,
alternate three pellets of each.
Depending on the cause, you may supplement with one of the following:
• bleeding caused by getting hit on the nose,
ARNICA MONTANA 9 C.
• nosebleed during a headache,
BELLADONNA 9 C.
• nosebleed during fever,
FERRUM PHOSPHORICUM 9 C.

Blood in urine:
CANTHARIS 5 C.

Uterus (bleeding between menstrual periods):
CINCHONA OFFICINALIS 5 C.
See your gynecologist.

Blennorrhagia

A discharge from mucous surfaces, usually the urethra or vagina.

Like most infectious diseases, blennorrhagia caused by infection could be treated using Homeopathy. But since gonorrhea is often the cause and is so easily transmitted through sexual contact, antibiotics, which act faster than homeopathic medicines, are used as the first line of treatment. Sometimes the surface of a baby's eyes will be infected at birth by passage through a vagina infected by gonorrhea, or in some cases, by another germ called chlamydia. Once the necessary antibiotics have been given, it is essential for a homeopathic doctor to determine a long-term preventive treatment to avoid negative aftereffects. Antibiotics alone can't correct all the effects following infection of the organism.

Blepharitis

Inflammation of the eyelid.

▷ *See* **Eyelids.**

Blisters

For blisters on the palm of the hand or on the heel, use:
CANTHARIS 9 C,
three pellets three times a day.

Apply CALENDULA ointment locally twice daily.

Bloatedness

To prevent fermentation and the production of gas by digestive bacteria, take three pellets of the following medicines three times a day:

Depending on localization:
- bloatedness of the stomach,
  CARBO VEGETABILIS 9 C.
- bloatedness in the lower area of the chest,
  LYCOPODIUM CLAVATUM 9 C.
- generalized bloatedness of the stomach and abdomen,
  CINCHONA OFFICINALIS 9 C.

Depending on the accompanying symptoms:
- bloatedness with a feeling of constriction in the pit of the stomach,
  CARBO VEGETABILIS 9 C.
- bloatedness accompanied by shortness of breath,
  CARBO VEGETABILIS 9 C.
- bloatedness accompanied by fatigue after meals,
  NUX VOMICA 9 C.

Depending on what relieves it:
- bloatedness relieved by bringing up air,
  CARBO VEGETABILIS 9 C.
- bloatedness relieved by passing gas,
  LYCOPODIUM CLAVATUM 9 C.

Depending on the cause:
- bloatedness due to nervousness,
  VALERIANA OFFICINALIS 9 C.
- bloatedness during menstrual periods,
  COCCULUS INDICUS 9 C.
- bloatedness after childbirth,
  SEPIA 9 C.

If you have difficulty choosing between any two of the above-mentioned medicines, alternate three pellets of each three times a day.

Blood (Diseases of)

Major blood diseases, such as leukemia, are not within the realm of Homeopathy. Some homeopathic treatments, however, can serve as auxiliary therapy to make the patient feel more comfortable. Ask your doctor.

Blows

▷ *See* **Injuries.**

Blushing

PULSATILLA 9 C,
three pellets three times a day for a period of several months will reduce the frequency of this emotional manifestation.

Boils (Furuncles)

Check with your doctor.

▷ *See* **Abscess.**

Bones

Decalcification, osteoporosis, and osteomyelitis may be treated by a homeopathic physician. A consultation is advisable.

▷ *Also see* **Demineralization, Fractures, Rheumatism.**

Borax

Base substance: Sodium borate.

Characteristic signs and symptoms: Painful mouth sores that tend to bleed; the mouth feels hot; fear of downward movements (the child begins to cry when lowered toward his or her bed).

Main clinical uses:
Aphthae (mouth sores).
Thrush and the problems caused for breast-feeding: *WARNING - This disease is serious. Contact your physician immediately for treatment recommendation.*

Brain concussion

▷ *See* **Trauma** (head).

Breast-feeding

Breast-feeding is the ideal. Formula feeding should be a last resort, only if the mother has been told by her doctor not to breast-feed her baby, or if separation of the mother and baby is unavoidable.

Fortunately, there is a general revival of interest in breast-feeding. Mother's milk is the only biological product that a baby is naturally ready for. The nutritive elements and natural antibodies in maternal milk will best enable a newborn to fight off infections. Maternal milk is also more easily digestible than formula. Small problems with breast-feeding may arise, which can be dealt with in the following ways:

Breast abscesses:
• Possible abscess; the breast feels hot and drawn,
    BRYONIA ALBA 9 C,
    three pellets three times a day.
• Early stages of abscess; the skin is red,
    BELLADONNA 9 C,
    three pellets three times a day.
• Abscess with pus,
    HEPAR SULPHURIS CALCAREUM 9 C,
    three pellets three times a day.

Apply CALENDULA M.T. locally—twenty-five drops on a frequently-changed compress.

Engorgement of the breasts:
    BRYONIA ALBA 9 C,
    three pellets three times a day.

Fatigue due to breast-feeding:
    CINCHONA OFFICINALIS 9 C,
    three pellets three times a day.

Insufficient milk supply:
    URTICA URENS 9 C,
    three pellets three times a day.

Overabundant milk supply:
    PULSATILLA 9 C,
    three pellets three times a day.

Painful breasts while feeding:
    PHELLANDRIUM AQUATICUM 9 C,
    three pellets ten minutes before feeding.

For weaning:
    RICINUS 30 C,
    one unit-dose tube per day taken by the mother for three days will stop milk production.

Breasts

Take three pellets of the chosen remedy three times a day for the following conditions:

Minor abscess:
    HEPAR SULPHURIS CALCAREUM 9 C.

Breast-feeding:
▷ *see* this entry.

Atrophy:
    IODIUM 5 C.

Cancer:
▷ *see* this entry.

Cracks around the nipple:
    GRAPHITES 9 C.
    A local treatment may be necessary; consult a health professional.

Cosmetic surgery:
▷ *see* this entry.

Pain:
- from trauma to the breast,
  BELLIS PERENNIS 9 C.
- sudden pain when the breasts are touched,
  CONIUM MACULATUM 9 C.
- painful breasts before menstrual periods,
  CONIUM MACULATUM 9 C.
- painful breasts while nursing,
  PHELLANDRIUM AQUATICUM 9 C.

Sagging breasts:
CONIUM MACULATUM 9 C.

Swelling of the breasts before menstrual periods:
SEPIA 9 C.

Tightening sensation in the breasts before menstrual periods:
LAC CANINUM 9 C.

Inflammation (redness only, no pus):
PHYTOLACCA DECANDRA 9 C.

When young girls' breasts produce milk:
PULSATILLA 9 C.

Cysts, nodules or lumps:
- for an isolated nodule,
  CONIUM MACULATUM 9 C.
- for multiple nodules,
  PHYTOLACCA DECANDRA 9 C.

WARNING: Examine your breasts frequently, such as when you bathe or shower or dress in front of a mirror. Learn how to examine your breasts, with fingers flat, standing up and lying down, your arms down and up. Your doctor or gynecologist can show you, and will give you printed information about breast self-examination (BSE). Anytime you feel a lump in your breast or notice an unusual wrinkling of the skin, report it to your doctor or gynecologist. Many lumps are just cysts and aren't malignant—but all lumps need to be examined promptly.

Breath (Bad)

The best homeopathic remedy for bad breath is:
MERCURIUS SOLUBILIS 9 C,
three pellets three times a day or whenever you have problems with bad breath.

If the symptoms persist, consult a homeopathic doctor or dentist.

Breath-holding spell

Young children will occasionally hold their breath when upset in order to "bargain or blackmail" their parents into noticing them or giving them what they want. This occasionally goes to extremes and the child loses consciousness for a short time from lack of oxygen. This type of behavior is usually harmless although it might be quite impressive to the parents at first. If your child seems to be prone to breath-holding spells, speak to your doctor or pediatrician (you need to make sure that the child doesn't have a real breathing problem), and give your child the following medicine: (By the way, these children start breathing on their own again once they get dizzy or black-out for a few moments).
IGNATIA AMARA 9 C,
three pellets three times a day, twenty days a month over a period of several months.

Bromium

Base substance: Bromine.

Characteristic signs and symptoms:
Chronic colds with the sensation of inhaling cold air; raucous cough; asthma accompanied by difficulty with

inhaling (and not exhaling, as is usually the case); asthma flaring up in sailors as soon as they return to land; hard lymph nodes; hardening of the thyroid.

Main clinical uses:
Chronic colds; hardened lymph nodes; firm goiter.
Asthma, laryngitis: *WARNING - These diseases are serious. Contact your physician immediately for treatment recommendation.*

Bronchial catarrh

Follow advice given for **Bronchitis.**

Bronchitis

Acute bronchitis

Antibiotics are not always absolutely necessary if acute bronchitis is correctly treated by Homeopathy. Here are a few treatments to choose from depending on the symptoms:

> HEPAR SULPHURIS CALCAREUM 9 C, three pellets to be taken without fail three times a day, plus one of the following, depending on the case:

- bronchitis with deep, congested sounds in the chest; a feeling of being suffocated by mucus; drowsiness,
> ANTIMONIUM TARTARICUM 9 C, three pellets three times a day.
- bronchitis with wheezing in the chest,
> IPECAC 9 C, three pellets three times a day.
- bronchitis with a small, dry cough,
> BRYONIA ALBA 9 C, three pellets three times a day.

- bronchitis with large lumps of yellow phlegm,
> MERCURIUS SOLUBILIS 9 C, three pellets three times a day.
- bronchitis with lumps of stringy greenish-yellow phlegm,
> KALI BICHROMICUM 9 C, three pellets three times a day.

If the treatment seems to be working after 48 hours, continue it for ten days. If not, consult a physician.

Chronic bronchitis

Chronic bronchitis and recurring bronchitis can both be treated by Homeopathy. When a person has suffered from bronchitis for a long time, however, there may be damage to the bronchial cartilages and pulmonary cavities.
In this case, you should consult a homeopathic physician for an in-depth constitutional treatment. This is especially important for infants and children.

Bryonia alba

Base substance: White bryony.

Characteristics signs and symptoms:
Sharp pains (in the head, lumbar region, around the liver, in the joints, etc.); dryness of the mucous membranes; intense thirst; dry cough; a sensation as if there were a stone in the stomach; constipation due to dryness of the rectum; damage to the joint ligaments; water on the joint; dizziness at the slightest movement; fever accompanied by a desire to remain still; symptoms aggravated by the slightest movement and relieved by external pressure.

Main clinical uses:
Flu-like symptoms with fever, intense thirst, fatigue, body aches; migraine

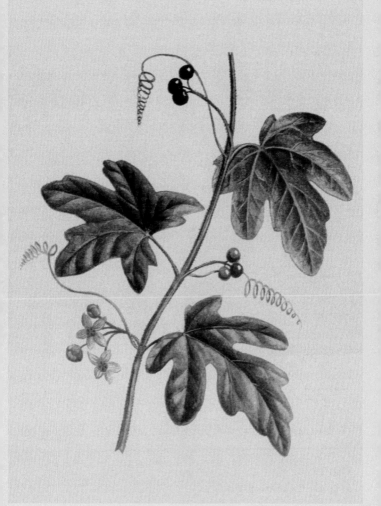

Bryonia alba

headaches; dizziness; rheumatism; lumbago; relief of symptoms of gallstones; constipation; a sharp pain in the side; pleurisy; breast abscess; hydrarthrosis ("water on the joint") or abundant flow of synovial fluid in a joint cavity.

WARNING: If condition worsens or persists for more than 72 hours, check with your physician.

Bulimia

• To control the appetite of a regular big-eater,
  ANTIMONIUM CRUDUM 9 C,
  three pellets three times a day.
• To calm a bout of nervous overeating caused by anxiety,
  IGNATIA AMARA 9 C,
  three pellets three times a day.
• For people who eat constantly but still lose weight,
  NATRUM MURIATICUM 9 C,
  same dosage.

Bunions

You may treat bunions (swelling of the joint of the big toe) with:
  APIS MELLIFICA 9 C,
  three pellets three times a day.

Apply HYPERICUM PERFORATUM M.T. locally once a day.

An operation to set the big toe right again may only be required when the malformation is very noticeable ("hallux valgus") or very painful.

Burns

▷ *See* **Injuries, Stomach, Sun.**

C

Cactus grandiflorus

Base substance: Night-blooming cereus.

Characteristic signs and symptoms:
A somewhat generalized sensation of constriction, especially around the heart, which feels like it were in a vise; strong palpitations; a tendency to bleed.

Main clinical uses:
Anxiety causing pains in the heart; various forms of neuralgia.

WARNING: You must see your doctor for any severe chest pain.

Calcarea carbonica

Base substance: Calcium carbonate from the middle layer of the oyster shell.

Suitable for:
People with a round head, pale complexion, and square teeth. Their limbs are short and when held out to their sides can't be extended high enough to form a 180° angle; children with growth retardation, particularly with late-closing fontanelles; children with learning difficulties.

Characteristic signs and symptoms:
Localized cold sensations; sweaty head and feet; a craving for eggs; acidity in the digestive tract; clay-like stools; profuse menstrual flow and periods brought on by minor emotional upsets; rashes on the scalp; swollen lymph nodes; catching cold easily.

Main clinical uses:
Rickets, biliary colic (gallstones), renal colic (kidney stones): _WARNING - These diseases are serious. Contact your physician immediately for treatment recommendation._

Acidic diarrhea; impetigo of newborns; anemia; polyps; repeated upper respiratory infections.

Calcarea fluorica

Base substance: Calcium fluoride.

Suitable for:
People with asymmetric bodies, misaligned teeth, and loose limbs that when fully extended form an angle greater than 180°.

Characteristic signs and symptoms:
Elastic-like muscle and joint tissues; varicose veins; a tendency to bony knots; induration of the tissues of lymph nodes, bones, genital organs, and the skin.

Main clinical uses:
Rickets: _WARNING - This disease is serious. Contact your physician immediately for treatment recommendation._
Varicose ulcers; varicose veins.

Calcarea phosphorica

Base substance: Calcium phosphate.

Suitable for:
Tall people with rectangular teeth that are longer than wide, and long limbs that form a 180° angle when stretched out to the sides.

Characteristic signs and symptoms:
Fragile bones; headaches from thinking; tendancy to catch cold easily (common cold, rhinopharyngitis, tonsillitis, inflammation of the lungs, etc.); swollen lymph nodes; green diarrhea with foul-smelling gas; anal fistula; phosphates in the urine.

Main clinical uses:
Anemia and rickets: _WARNING - These diseases are serious. Contact_

your physician immediately for treatment recommendation.
Fractures; repeated infection of the upper respiratory passages.

Calculi (Stones)

Gallstones or kidney stones.

Homeopathy cannot dissolve these stones, but it can help reduce the pain and prevent complications of infection.
Surgical removal of a stone may be necessary when:
• a gallstone gets lodged in the bile duct.
• a kidney stone gets lodged in one of the ureters or in the kidney.
It may be possible to avoid an operation in other instances if you adhere to homeopathic treatment. Consult a homeopathic physician to find out the best treatment course.

▷ *Also see* **Colic** (biliary and renal).

Calendula officinalis

Base substance: Common or garden pot marigold.
Characteristic signs and symptoms: Minor cuts and scrapes; the relief of minor skin irritations due to cuts, abrasions or skin conditions.
Main clinical use: Local application of the "Mother-Tincture," ointment, or lotion on wounds.

Camphor

Camphor is a neutralizing agent or **antidote** (see this entry) to all forms of homeopathic medicines.

Camphora

Base substance: Camphor.
Suitable for: Effects of cold.
Characteristic signs and symptoms: After exposure to the cold, the skin is cold to the touch, the breath is cold but the patient refuses to be covered up; lack of strength; muscle cramps; abundant diarrhea and decreased urine.
Main clinical uses: Onset of a severe chill; the common cold.

Cancer

Cancer treatments are beyond the realm of Homeopathy. However, a few well-chosen homeopathic medicines can help the patient feel more comfortable and help prevent some of the complications of infection. Consult a homeopathic physician.

Candidiasis (Yeast infections)

Candidiasis is an inflammation of the mucous membranes, particularly of the mouth, intestinal tract, or vagina, caused by the yeast "Candida albicans."
For this disease, you must consult your physician.

Cantharis

Base substance: Spanish fly.
Characteristic signs and symptoms: A frequent urge to pass water accompanied by painful urination; blood in the urine; urinating drop by

drop (dribbling); heightened sexual interest; intense thirst without being able to drink; large blisters on the skin.

Main clinical uses:
Cystitis, diarrhea accompanied by a urinary tract infection: *WARNING - These diseases are serious. Contact your physician immediately for treatment recommendation.*
Skin burns with blisters: *WARNING - If condition worsens or persists for more than 72 hours, check with your physician.*

Capillaries (Dilated facial)

Dilation of the superficial facial capillaries and small blood vessels; the process cannot usually be reversed but may be halted with:
CARBO ANIMALIS 9 C,
three pellets three times a day, twenty days a month.

Capsicum annuum

Base substance: Garden pimento, also known as Red pepper.

Characteristic signs and symptoms:
A burning sensation of the mucous membranes, particularly the throat (as if one had swallowed a red pepper); sore throat with pains radiating to the ears; inflammation of the mastoids; intense thirst; shivering when drinking liquids.

Main clinical uses:
Mastoiditis, otitis: *WARNING - These diseases are serious. Contact your physician immediately for treatment recommendation.*
Sore throat.

Carbo vegetabilis

Base substance: Vegetable or wood charcoal.

Characteristic signs and symptoms:
Stagnation of the blood circulation; congestion in the veins; shortness of breath; desire for fresh air and desire to be fanned; bloating of the stomach accompanied by constrictive pains; difficulty digesting fats; warm-feeling head and cool body; hoarseness, particularly in the evening; worn-out feeling.

Main clinical uses:
Poor digestion; dyspepsia; distension of the abdomen above the navel; flatulence; aerophagia (air swallowing); asthma; circulatory disorders; migraines; onset of cough.

WARNING: If condition worsens or persists for more than 72 hours, check with your physician.

Carduus marianus

Base substance: St. Mary's thistle, also known as Milk thistle.

Characteristic signs and symptoms:
Pain and increase in volume of the left side of the liver; bilious vomiting; constipation; sallow skin; varicose ulcers; dizziness.

Main clinical uses:
Hepatitis, gallstones (biliary colic): *WARNING - These diseases are serious. Contact your physician immediately for treatment recommendation.*
Hepatic insufficiency.

Carsickness

▷ See **Travel sickness.**

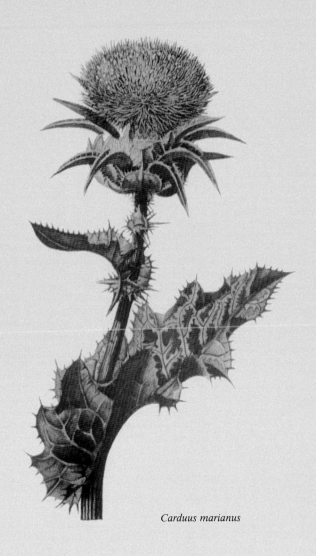

Carduus marianus

Cataracts

▷ *See* **Eyes.**

Caulophyllum thalictroides

Base substance: Blue cohosh.

Characteristic signs and symptoms:
Delay of progression of labor due to cervical rigidity, false contractions; menstrual pains that mimic contractions.

Main clinical uses:
Painful menstrual periods.
Facilitation of childbirth: *WARNING - Contact your physician for treatment recommendation.*

Cause of Illnesses

The cause of an illness can help determine the appropriate homeopathic treatment.
When the cause of a disease is known, it's easier for the physician to prescribe a suitable medicine. For example, the signs and symptoms of distress suggest treatment with IGNATIA AMARA, NATRUM MURIATICUM, or PHOSPHORICUM ACIDUM. This does not mean, however, that the homeopathic doctor automatically prescribes one, or all three, of these medicines. He or she questions and examines the patient first, and studies all the symptoms before coming to a decision. Finding "causality," as homeopaths call it, speeds up finding the appropriate medicine. But this is not true in every case, and it may happen that the doctor will prescribe a drug other than one of the three mentioned above. The art of practicing homeopathic medicine requires patience.
It's not always possible to identify the cause or causes of an illness, yet **not finding a cause does not rule out a treatment.** The patient's symptoms and the Law of Similars enables the homeopathic doctor to find the necessary individualized therapy. Knowing the cause of an illness is always preferable, but is not indispensable for proper homeopathic treatment.

Causticum

Base substance: A preparation derived from caustic lime and potassium bisulphate.

Suitable for:
Sad, depressed people who are easily influenced by the unhappiness of others, and who are apprehensive of imminent danger.

Characteristic signs and symptoms:
Localized chronic paralysis which sets in slowly and progressively, especially after the patient has been exposed to a dry, cold environment; stiffness and deformation of the joints which is improved by a humid environment; a burning sensation of the mucous membranes; passing urine while coughing; sallow, dry skin; large warts that bleed easily; old, painful scars.

Main clinical uses:
Paralysis, in particular of the face; urinary incontinence: *WARNING - These diseases are serious. Contact your physician immediately for treatment recommendation.*
Warts; deforming rheumatism; constipation; laryngitis.

Ceanothus americanus

Base substance: New Jersey tea.

Suitable for: Aftereffects of malaria.

Characteristic signs and symptoms:
Painful, enlarged spleen; diarrhea.

Main clinical use:
Troubles of the spleen: _WARNING -
This disease is serious. Contact your
physician immediately for treatment
recommendation._

Cedron

Base substance: Cedrone.

Characteristic signs and symptoms:
Pain in the forehead, going from one
temple to the other; fever with
numbness of the limbs; regular return
of the symptoms (they always come
back at the same time each day).

Main clinical uses:
Migraine; facial neuralgia.

Celiac disease

▷ _See_ **Gluten intolerance.**

Cell Salts (Schuessler's)

According to the biochemic theory of
Dr. W. H. Schuessler (a German
physician who practiced in the 1870's),
there are twelve mineral compounds
(or cell salts) that are needed by the
body in minute quantities to nourish
and strengthen certain cells.
Deficiencies in any one of these salts
can create symptoms of illness which
vary according to the specific salt that
is lacking. The body's defense
mechanisms usually keep the body

cells naturally in balance; however,
improper diet and processed food, lack
of exercise and modern-day stress can
create a tissue salt imbalance or
deficiency. Through use of the
appropriate biochemic tissue remedies
in an assimilable form, the cells are
brought back into proper balance,
resulting in normal body functions.
Each mineral salt is prepared
according to the methods described by
Schuessler and the stringent standards
of the Homeopathic Pharmacopeia of
the United States. The potentized
triturations of these 12 Cell Salts are
used, along with the indicated
homeopathic treatment, as nutritional
supplements to insure optimal health
maintenance.

Cephalea

▷ _See_ **Headache.**

Chalazion (Stye)

▷ _See_ **Eyelids.**

Chamomile

▷ _See_ **Antidotes.**

Chamomilla

Base substance: Camomile or
Chamomile.

Suitable for:
Ill-tempered children who are restless
and squeamish, often with one red
cheek and one pale cheek.

Characteristic signs and symptoms:
Poor toleration to pain, apparently
relieved when the child is carried or

pushed in the stroller; hot sweating from the head; green diarrhea; restlessness; bad temper.

Main clinical uses:
Teething problems with pain, irritability and fever; facial neuralgia; menstrual pains; insomnia; rheumatism; diarrhea; nervousness in children.

<u>*WARNING:*</u> *If condition worsens or persists for more than 72 hours, check with your physician.*

Change of life

▷ *See* **Menopause.**

Chapping

▷ *See* **Cracks of the skin.**

Character (Personality)

Homeopathy can't change a person's personality. But it can help to subdue extremes in character and certain personality traits that make life difficult for the patient or those around him.
Certain character traits can indicate which therapy is most suitable. Combined with symptoms, they will help the physician decide on the appropriate course of treatment. For example, a shy girl easily prone to tears and who needs much consolation and affection automatically makes the physician think of PULSATILLA. This medicine will relieve poor circulation, aid digestion, and make her feel less like crying so often. She will remain, however, a sensitive person.

▷ *Also see* **Typology.**

Cheeks

Desquamation: ▷ *see* this entry.
Red cheeks: ▷ *see* **Capillaries.**

Cheiranthus cheiri

Base substance: Gillyflower.
Main clinical use: Inflammation of wisdom teeth.

Chelidonium majus

Base substance: Celandine, also known as Tetter-wort.

Chelidonium majus

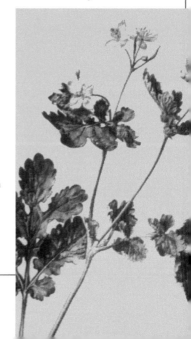

Characteristic signs and symptoms:
Pain in the region of the gallbladder;
pain in the lower edge of the right
shoulder blade; enlarged liver; sallow
skin; eyes tinged with yellow;
dark-colored urine; colorless stools
that float; itching of the anus;
headache.

Main clinical uses:
Spasms or inflammation of the bile
ducts; rheumatism.
Hepatitis; jaundice; pulmonary
disorders accompanied by bilious
complications; migraines: *WARNING
- These diseases are serious. Contact
your physician immediately for
treatment recommendation.*

Cheloma

Hypertrophied or badly-healed scars.

▷ See **Scars.**

Chemicals

So-called chemical medicines: ▷ *see*
Allopathy.

*Are chemical products used in
Homeopathy?* ▷ *see* **Allopathy.**

Chickenpox

A childhood disease that can usually
be treated at home (small vesicles all
over the body, accompanied by fever).

WARNING: Check with your doctor.
Once the diagnosis has been
determined, take:
  ANTIMONIUM TARTARICUM 9 C,
  RHUS TOXICODENDRON 9 C,
  SULPHUR 9 C,
  alternate three pellets of each,
  three times a day for six days.

Chilblains

Redness and pain of the extremities
(hands, feet), generally due to the cold
(frostbite). Never try to ease the pain
by immediately putting your hands
into warm water. Cool tap water and
one of the medicines below will help
dispel discomfort.

*WARNING: Severe frostbite should be
seen by your doctor.*

General treatment

Take three pellets of one of the
following medicines three times a day,
depending on the circumstances:

If the chilblains are aggravated by:
● heat,
  AGARICUS MUSCARIUS 9 C,
  PULSATILLA 9 C.
● being touched,
  NITRICUM ACIDUM 9 C,

If they are improved by:
● cool temperatures,
  APIS MELLIFICA 9 C,
● warmth (gradual),
  ARSENICUM ALBUM 9 C.

Depending on the color:
● if the skin is red,
  AGARICUS MUSCARIUS 9 C.
● if it's pink,
  APIS MELLIFICA 9 C.
● if it's almost black,
  ARSENICUM ALBUM 9 C.
● if it's purple,
  PULSATILLA 9 C.

Depending on the sensations:
● chilblains that feel like icy needles,
  AGARICUS MUSCARIUS 9 C.
● itchy chilblains,
  RHUS TOXICODENDRON 9 C.

*Depending on symptoms occurring at
the same time:*
● chilblains accompanied by skin
ulcerations,
  NITRICUM ACIDUM 9 C.
● chilblains with cracks in the skin,
  PETROLEUM 9 C.

A **local treatment** could be a good complement. Apply CALENDULA ointment directly on affected areas.

Childbirth

WARNING: Check with your doctor.

With Homeopathy, childbirth can be experienced with as little pain as possible and under the best psychological conditions.

Preparing for delivery:
- To ease the fear of giving birth,
  CIMICIFUGA RACEMOSA 12 C,
  one unit-dose tube every week during the ninth month.
- To make contractions more effective and speed up delivery,
  CAULOPHYLLUM 12 C,
  one unit-dose tube every week during the ninth month.
- To avoid the physical trauma which may be associated with childbirth, and maintain the strength necessary to deliver the baby,
  ARNICA MONTANA 12 C,
  one unit-dose tube every week during the ninth month.

It is recommended that you take one unit-dose tube of the above medicines every week during the last month of pregnancy, spreading them out as follows:

CIMICIFUGA RACEMOSA on Monday,
CAULOPHYLLUM on Wednesday,
ARNICA MONTANA on Friday.

During the delivery, your doctor may prescribe:
- In case of strong, ineffective contractions,
  NUX VOMICA 5 C,
  BELLADONNA 5 C,
  alternate three pellets of each, every five minutes.
- If the baby is overdue (the due date is past),

GELSEMIUM SEMPERVIRENS 9 C,
three pellets every hour.
- In case of fatigue or exhaustion,
  ARNICA MONTANA 9 C,
  three pellets every hour (if this remedy hasn't been taken preventively).

After the delivery:
- For post-natal depression,
  SEPIA 9 C,
  three pellets three times a day.
- For fatigue or lumbar pains,
  KALI CARBONICUM 9 C,
  three pellets three times a day.
- For post-natal pains in the abdomen,
  ARNICA MONTANA 9 C,
  three pellets three times a day.
- For persistent vaginal bleeding,
  (Check with your doctor.)
  HAMAMELIS VIRGINICA 9 C,
  three pellets three times a day.
- For white discharge streaked with blood from the vagina, (Check with your doctor.)
  CREOSOTUM 9 C,
  three pellets three times a day.

▷ *Also see* **Breast-feeding, Pregnancy.**

Children (Childhood diseases)

▷ For specific childhood diseases, look up the corresponding headings, such as **German measles, Mumps, Chickenpox,** etc.

WARNING: You should always seek your doctor's advice promptly when faced with a young child who looks or acts differently, or seems really sick—unusual paleness, unusual tiredness, unusual irritability. Only the doctor has the necessary competence to judge the situation and prescribe an appropriate treatment course.

Homeopathic treatments often work well with children. The medicines act

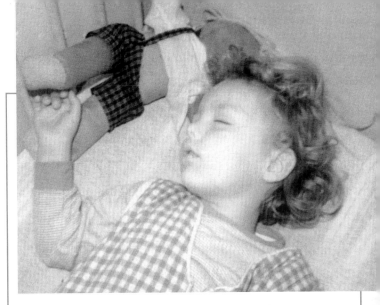

A child without problems, peacefully asleep.

A child suffering from insomnia. How can you tell if your child is just pretending or is really upset about something?

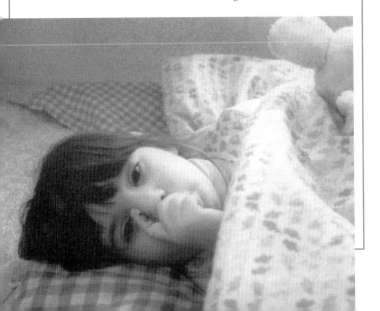

rapidly and, because of their pleasant taste, are readily accepted by children. Some homeopaths specialize in pediatric Homeopathy.

It is important to keep in mind that the recommended doses of homeopathic medicines are always the same for all ages—children as well as adults. What counts with homeopathic treatment isn't the amount of active substance in a homeopathic medicine, but the presence of the right substance itself.

For a nervous child, select one of the medicines below and give three pellets three times a day for several weeks. Consult a homeopathic physician if nervousness or anxiety are chronic in your child's behavior.

Restlessness:
- while teething,
  CHAMOMILLA 9 C.
- for a child who can't sit still,
  TARENTULA HISPANICA 9 C.
- fears not being loved any more,
  PULSATILLA 9 C.
- dislikes being bathed,
  ANTIMONIUM CRUDUM 9 C.
- for stuttering,
  STRAMONIUM 9 C.
- for sulking,
  NATRUM MURIATICUM 9 C.
- tends toward moodiness,
  CHAMOMILLA 9 C.
- tends toward anger,
  NUX VOMICA 9 C.
- for the child who lacks confidence but still does well at school,
  SILICEA 9 C.
- for cruelty (toward animals, other children); the child enjoys making others suffer,
  MERCURIUS SOLUBILIS 9 C.
- for squeamishness; the child is afraid of the slightest pain,
  CHAMOMILLA 9 C.
- plays with fire,
  HEPAR SULPHURIS CALCAREUM 9 C.
- for the child who is grumpy,
  ANTIMONIUM CRUDUM 9 C.

- for the imaginative child who fantasizes inappropriately,
  SULPHUR 9 C.

Irritability:
- constant irritability,
  CHAMOMILLA 9 C.
- when suffering from worms,
  CINCHONA OFFICINALIS 9 C.
- at the seaside, on the beach,
  NATRUM MURIATICUM 9 C.

Jealousy:
  HYOSCYAMUS NIGER 9 C.

Making fun of others:
  HYOSCYAMUS NIGER 9 C.

Fear of new people or things ("stranger anxiety"); the child hides when visitors come:
  LYCOPODIUM CLAVATUM 9 C.

Fear:
- if the child is afraid of intruders,
  NATRUM MURIATICUM 9 C.
- of the dark,
  STRAMONIUM 9 C.

Cries for no reason:
  PULSATILLA 9 C.

Sleep-associated problems:
- if the child cries in his or her sleep,
  APIS MELLIFICA 9 C.
- can't get to sleep,
  BELLADONNA 9 C.
- sweats in their sleep,
  CALCAREA CARBONICA 9 C.
- sleepwalks,
  KALI BROMATUM 9 C.
- drools in their sleep,
  MERCURIUS SOLUBILIS 9 C.
- has fears at night, nightmares,
  STRAMONIUM 9 C.

Nervous tics:
  AGARICUS MUSCARIUS 9 C.

Wants to touch everything:
  CHAMOMILLA 9 C,

If the child wets his pants slightly from time to time during the day,
  PHOSPHORUS 9 C.

Chimaphila umbellata

Base substance: American wintergreen.

Characteristic signs and symptoms:
Large amounts of mucus in the urine; sensation of a ball in the perineum; difficult, forced urination.

Main clinical uses:
Inflammation of the bladder:
WARNING - This disease is serious. Contact your physician immediately for treatment recommendation.
Prostatic complications.

Chionanthus virginica

Base substance: Fringe tree.

Characteristic signs and symptoms:
Migraines with bilious vomiting; enlarged liver; enlarged spleen; sallow skin.

Main clinical uses: Recurrent migraines; jaundice.

WARNING: If condition worsens or persists for more than 72 hours, check with your physician.

Cholecystitis

Infection of the gallbladder. Check with your doctor.
Take:
    MERCURIUS SOLUBILIS 9 C,
    PYROGENIUM 9 C,
    alternate three pellets of each, three times a day.

WARNING: See a doctor if your complexion turns yellow, or if your fever does not disappear.

▷ *Also see* **Colic** (biliary), **Calculi (stones)**.

Cholera (Historical account of)

A virulent cholera epidemic hit New York in 1832. Both allopaths and homeopaths worked courageously to combat this acute infectious disease that terrorized the population and took its toll of lives. Rapidly, it became evident that the homeopaths were obtaining comparably better results; these results were such that conventional doctors were often willing to adopt homeopathic remedies. This was also true for the critical Cincinatti epidemic of 1849. Once the dreaded epidemics had subsided by the end of the century, homeopathic medicine had without a doubt gained considerable ground. As a consequence of its medical successes, Homeopathy had not only proved itself therapeutically effective but also had shown that it took interest in the patient as a human being. Compared to the bloodletting, purges and emetics which were common allopathic medicinal procedures, homeopathic treatment brought real affecting comfort to its patients; it was relief they had long been expecting.[1]
Traditionally, homeopathic physicians have treated cholera in the following manner:
• For the onset of cholera, with shock and sensation of cold,
    CAMPHORA 9 C.
• For a serious case with restlessness,
    ARSENICUM ALBUM 9 C.
• For severe cramps,
    CUPRUM METALLICUM 9 C.
• For diarrhea and cold sweats,
    VERATRUM ALBUM 9 C.

WARNING: This disease is serious.

---

1. Coulter, Harris L., *Divided Legacy*, Richmond, California: North Atlantic Books, 1973.

Cholesterol

Excess cholesterol in the blood is not the only form of fat or lipid disease. Doctors also place importance on the dangers of too many triglycerides. A change in diet, along with homeopathic medicines (PODOPHYLLUM PELTATUM, COLCHICUM AUTUMNALE, CHOLESTERINUM), can bring cholesterol and triglyceride levels back to normal. Consult your physician.

Chorea

"St. Vitus' Dance" or "Sydenham's Chorea." A disorder of the nervous system, usually associated with acute rheumatism, characterized by spasmodic, involuntary movements. A rarer disorder today due to proper treatment for the causative streptococcus bacteria.
Consult a homeopathic physician; other medicines exist.

Chronic (Illness)

The concept of "chronic illness" is very important in Homeopathy. When a person suffers repeated attacks of the same illness (e.g., asthma), just treating the symptoms each time is not enough. A long-term treatment to modify the underlying "explosive" chronic condition is required.
There is a definite connection between the concept of chronic illness and the notion of terrain (see **Terrain).**
Treating a chronic illness is the ideal domain of the homeopathic doctor, since each case needs to be carefully studied to be mastered.

Cicuta virosa

Base substance: Water Hemlock, also known as Cowbane.

Characteristic signs and symptoms: Many kinds of violent spasms; dilation of the pupils; childish behavior.

Main clinical use: Spasmodic affections.

WARNING: If condition worsens or persists for more than 72 hours, check with your physician.

Cimicifuga racemosa (or Actea racemosa)

Base substance: Black cohosh.

Suitable for: Women with gynecological problems.

Characteristic signs and symptoms: Period pains (the heavier the menstrual flow, the stronger the pain); throbbing menstrual migraines; intense muscular pains, especially in the back; moodiness; fear of childbirth; talkativeness; all of these symptoms appear to depend on the condition of the uterus and become worse during periods.

Main clinical uses: Painful periods; menstrual headaches; preparation for childbirth; disorders related to menopause; torticollis (wryneck); rheumatism.

Cina

Base substance: the Wormseed.

Suitable for: Children with worms; restless children who grind their teeth and have rings under their eyes.

Characteristic signs and symptoms:
Insatiable hunger; itching nose;
stomach pains especially around the
navel; coughing; itching in the anus;
nervous restlessness.

Main clinical uses:
Vermiculosis, or worm-infestation
(this product will stop the symptoms,
but not get rid of the worms):
*WARNING: If condition worsens or
persists for more than 72 hours, check
with your physician.*
Nervousness in children; cough.

Cinchona officinalis
(or China)

Base substance: China or Cinchona
bark.

Suitable for:
Anemia; fluid loss from bleeding,
vomiting or diarrhea; relapses of
malaria (acts on the symptoms, does
not kill the parasite).

Characteristic signs and symptoms:
Abdominal distension (bloating);
painless diarrhea that leaves the
patient feeling weak; enlarged liver;
enlarged spleen; a pattern of fever
every other day; bleeding of
dark-colored blood; nosebleeds;
sensitivity to touch and light; ringing
in the ears; throbbing headaches;
rheumatism with swelling of the joints;
weakness; periodic return of the
symptoms.

Main clinical uses:
Indigestion; painless diarrhea that
leaves the patient feeling tired;

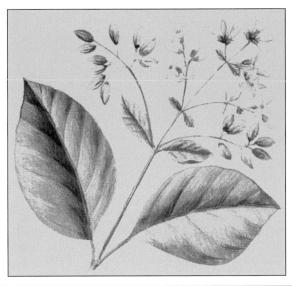

*Cinchona
officinalis*

61

rheumatism; fatigue caused by breast-feeding; aftereffects of bleeding or anemia leaving the patient feeling weak; nosebleeds; various kinds of fever; fatigue.

WARNING: If condition worsens or persists for more than 72 hours, check with your physician.

Circulation (Problems of)

Circulatory disorders are within the realm of Homeopathy.

▷ *See* the various headings concerned, in particular: **Menstrual periods, Phlebitis, Raynaud's Disease, Ulcers, Varicose veins.**

Cirrhosis (Fibrosis of the liver)

There is a homeopathic treatment for cirrhosis as long as it hasn't reached an irreversible, "decompensated," advanced stage.
For cirrhosis due to alcohol ingestion, the first thing is to stop drinking. The second is to consult a homeopathic physician who will prescribe an appropriate treatment. PHOSPHORUS will probably be one of the main elements prescribed.

▷ *Also see* **Alcoholism.**

Cistus canadensis

Base substance: Frost-weed.
Characteristic signs and symptoms: Catching cold from slight exposure to cold air; a sensation of cold inside the nose; chronic rhinitis; cervical lymph node swelling.
Main clinical uses: Colds; pharyngitis; swollen lymph nodes.

Claustrophobia

A fear of closed-in places. This can be treated with:
ARGENTUM NITRICUM 9 C,
three pellets three times a day, for two weeks a month over a period of several months.

Cocculus indicus

Base substance: Indian cockle.
Characteristic signs and symptoms: Dizziness caused by watching moving objects (cars, for example); headache (in the back of the skull) with the feeling that something is opening and closing there; painful muscular numbness; slowed movements; slowed thought processes.
Main clinical uses:
Attacks of hyperventilation:
WARNING - This disease is serious. You should consult your physician for advice.
Motion sickness with nausea and dizziness; insomnia due to stress; migraines; painful menstrual periods:
WARNING: If condition worsens or persists for more than 72 hours, check with your physician.

Coccus cacti

Base substance: Cochineal.
Characteristic signs and symptoms: Inflammation of the mucous membranes; coughing with large amounts of thick mucus which is difficult to expel; a tickling feeling in the larynx.
Main clinical uses: Spasmodic cough; laryngitis.

Coccyx (Tailbone)

For pains in the coccyx, take three pellets of one of the following remedies three times a day:
- For a fall on your coccyx,
  HYPERICUM PERFORATUM 9 C.
- For pain after being annoyed,
  IGNATIA AMARA 9 C.
- For a sensation of numbness in the tailbone,
  PLATINUM METALLICUM 9 C.

Coffea cruda

Base substance: Unroasted coffee beans.

Characteristic signs and symptoms:
Insomnia caused by a mind too full of ideas; incessant mental activity; physical restlessness; palpitations; intolerable pains.

Main clinical uses:
Insomnia; restlessness due to exhaustion or overexcitability; nervous heart; toothache.

<u>WARNING:</u> *If condition worsens or persists for more than 72 hours, check with your physician.*

Coffee

There are two main kinds of coffee:
- *Arabica,* which grows in South America,
- *Robusta,* which grows in Africa.
Robusta contains more caffeine than Arabica. For this reason it's wiser to drink pure Arabica whenever there is a choice and if you can't do without coffee completely. Arabica is more expensive than Robusta, so the two coffees are often blended.

Drinking too much coffee,
NUX VOMICA 9 C,
three pellets three times a day will help reduce intake.

Coffee

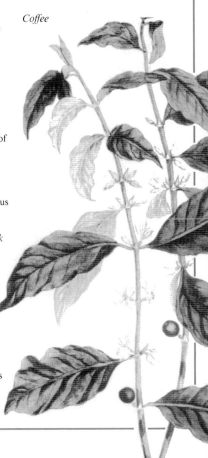

Dislike of the smell of coffee,
    IGNATIA AMARA 9 C,
    three pellets three times a day
    taken as long as the aversion lasts.

Muscle cramps caused by coffee,
    NUX VOMICA 9 C,
    three pellets three times a day.

Diarrhea caused by coffee,
    THUJA OCCIDENTALIS 9 C,
    three pellets three times a day.

Insomnia due to coffee,
    COFFEA CRUDA 9 C,
    three pellets every fifteen minutes
    until you fall asleep.

Headaches due to coffee,
    NUX VOMICA 9 C,
    three pellets three times a day.

Palpitations caused by coffee,
    NUX VOMICA 9 C,
    three pellets three times a day.

Colchicum autumnale

Base substance: Wild or meadow
saffron.

Characteristic signs and symptoms:
Acute attack of gout with joint redness
and extreme pain to touch; the attack
quickly moves from one joint to the
next; nausea caused by the smell of
food; recurrent autumnal diarrhea.

Main clinical uses:
Diarrhea, gout: *WARNING - These
diseases are serious. Contact your
physician immediately for treatment
recommendation.*

Cold (Tendency to catch)

To reduce a tendency to catch cold,
take:
    TUBERCULINUM NOSODE 30 C,
    one unit-dose tube per week for
    one or two months every winter.

▷ *Also see* **Cold sensitivity, Winter.**

Colds

At the slightest sign of a cold, take:
    INFLUENZINUM 30 C,
    one unit-dose tube as soon as
    symptoms occur.
    Alternate ACONITUM NAPELLUS 9 C
    with BRYONIA ALBA 9 C,
    three pellets of each three times a
    day.

If the cold is well-established, take
three pellets of one of the following
remedies three times a day:
- for clear, watery nasal discharge,
    ALLIUM CEPA 9 C.
- for nasal discharge of lumpy yellow
mucus,
    HYDRASTIS CANADENSIS 9 C.
- for greenish-yellow nasal discharge,
    KALI BICHROMICUM 9 C.
- for crusting in the nose,
    KALI BICHROMICUM 9 C.
- for yellow, irritating discharge,
    MERCURIUS SOLUBILIS 9 C.
- if you sneeze a great deal,
    NUX VOMICA 9 C.
- if your nose is stopped up at night
and runny during the day,
    NUX VOMICA 9 C.
- for yellow, non-irritating nasal
discharge,
    PULSATILLA 9 C.
- for loss of sense of taste and smell
while suffering from a cold,
    PULSATILLA 9 C.
- if the nose is stopped up and dry,
    SAMBUCUS NIGRA 9 C.

For recurring colds, check with a
doctor. While waiting, take:
    NATRUM MURIATICUM 9 C,
    three pellets three times a day.

Cold sensitivity

Cold sensitivity may indicate that the
body has trouble adjusting to cold
temperatures or that the blood is
circulating poorly. There are many
causes for cold intolerance and it is

difficult to outline therapeutic advice in such a short space. If you suffer from cold sensitivity, it would be better to check with a doctor. You may also try the following treatment:

PSORINUM 30 C,
one unit-dose tube a week for two or three months—provided you have no history of eczema.

Colic

Colic means "spasmodic pain," usually in the abdomen.

Abdominal colic (intestinal spasms):
COLOCYNTHIS 9 C,
MAGNESIA PHOSPHORICA 9 C,
alternate these two remedies every 15 minutes until pain has stopped.

Biliary or hepatic colic (spasms of the bile ducts, often touched off by stones):
BERBERIS VULGARIS 9 C,
CALCAREA CARBONICA 9 C,
MAGNESIA PHOSPHORICA 9 C,
alternate these three remedies every five minutes or every quarter of an hour, depending on intensity of pain. Take three pellets each time.

Renal colic (spasms of the urinary ducts, stones):
Dissolve five pellets of each of the following medicines in a large glass of water:

ARNICA MONTANA 9 C,
BELLADONNA 9 C,
BERBERIS VULGARIS 9 C,
CALCAREA CARBONICA 9 C,
LYCOPODIUM CLAVATUM 9 C,
OCIMUM CANUM 9 C,
PAREIRA BRAVA 9 C.

Stir well and take one teaspoonful every 15 minutes depending on intensity of pain.

WARNING: In any case, as with all serious conditions, consult your physician.

▷ Also see **Calculi.**

Colitis

Inflammation of the colon often with spasms and diverticulae (small outpouchings). The main symptoms are alternating diarrhea and constipation with abdominal pain. It is indispensable to have a homeopathic physician prescribe a long-term preventive treatment as well as a special diet. In the meantime, alternate three pellets of the following remedies three times a day:

NATRUM SULPHURICUM 9 C,
MAGNESIA PHOSPHORICA 9 C,
THUJA OCCIDENTALIS 9 C.

WARNING: In any case, as with all serious conditions, consult your physician.

Collinsonia canadensis

Base substance: Horse-weed, also known as Stone-root.

Characteristic signs and symptoms: Severe constipation, particularly during pregnancy; hemorrhoids which bleed with the sensation of being pricked by needles; hemorrhoids occurring with gynecological disorders; alternating hemorrhoids and palpitations, or hemorrhoids and headaches.

Main clinical uses: Constipation; hemorrhoids; itching of the anus.

Colocynthis

Base substance: Bitter apple, also known as Bitter gourd.

Characteristic signs and symptoms: Violent cramp-like pains which are relieved by heat and strong pressure; irritability due to pain.

Main clinical uses:
Abdominal colic (abdominal cramps);
sciatica; facial neuralgia; painful
menstrual periods; colicky pains
associated with diarrhea.

_WARNING: If condition worsens or
persists for more than 72 hours, check
with your physician._

Combination formulae

Combination formulae are mixtures of
homeopathic medicines which are
prepared in advance. They offer
therapeutic action when the physician
is unable to decide on the specific,
appropriate remedy for a given case.
Although they aren't particularly
recommended for most prescriptions,
they may prove helpful in short-term
self-medication. Their action is
superficial and temporary.

Computers

Can computers become an everyday
part of homeopathic medicine?
Computers, no matter how
sophisticated they become, will never
replace the clinical skill and acumen of
an experienced homeopathic
physician. However, homeopathic
software, which is already available,
may be an excellent tool for storing
data. But how to best use that data to
come to proper conclusions about the
prevention and treatment of disease
will always demand a good clinician's
mind and observation skills.

Condylomata

Warts in the genital and anal region.
These can often be successfully

eliminated with:
>THUJA OCCIDENTALIS 5 C,
>NITRICUM ACIDUM 5 C,
>alternate three pellets of each,
>three times a day over a period of
>one or two months.

Congestion

Hepatic congestion: ▷ see **Liver.**

Lung congestion:
>INFLUENZINUM 9 C,
>PHOSPHORUS 9 C,
>HEPAR SULPHURIS CALCAREUM 9 C,
>alternate three pellets of each,
>three times a day.

_WARNING: If symptoms persist,
discontinue use of the above remedies
and consult your physician._

Venous congestion: ▷ see **Varicose
veins.**

Conium maculatum

Base substance: Poison hemlock, also
known as Spotted hemlock.

Suitable for: Trauma of the breasts
and other glands.

Characteristic signs and symptoms:
Dizziness when turning the head to
one side, relieved by closing the eyes;
inability to make a mental effort;
lacrimation (excess tear flow); various
types of paralysis with difficulty in
walking; intermittent flow of urine;
induration (hardening) and
hypertrophy of the lymph nodes,
breasts, ovaries or prostate.

Main clinical uses:
Dizziness.
Breast swelling, swollen lymph glands,
various types of paralysis: _WARNING
- These diseases are serious. Contact
your physician immediately for
treatment recommendation._

Conjunctivitis

▷ *See* **Eyes.**

Constipation

Many people are aware of the dangers of using laxatives that irritate the intestinal mucosa (particularly, laxatives made with phenolphtaleine). Homeopathy can offer some good alternate medicines for constipation.

Constipation in longtime sufferers: Check with a doctor. You'll have a better chance of positive results than with self-medication.

Conium maculatum

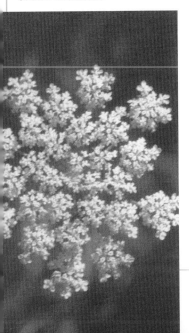

Recent constipation:
Take three pellets of the following remedies three times a day.
• If you need to push very hard to evacuate stools, even soft ones:
    ALUMINA 9 C.
• Colorless, light stools that float:
    CHELIDONIUM MAJUS 9 C.
• Large stools with strings of mucus:
    GRAPHITES 9 C.
• Constipation during menstrual periods:
    GRAPHITES 9 C.
• Constipation without the urge to defecate:
    HYDRASTIS CANADENSIS 9 C.
• Constipation during pregnancy or after childbirth:
    HYDRASTIS CANADENSIS 9 C.
• Constipation with the urge to defecate but being unable to:
    NUX VOMICA 9 C.
• Stools that are small and round like marbles:
    MAGNESIA MURIATICA 9 C.

Constitutions (Somatotypes)

▷ *See* **Typology.**

Continence

For disorders related to chastity, virginity, celibacy:

▷ *see* **Sexual disorders.**

Contraception

The doctor's role in this sensitive decision is to inform but not to decide. The choice is up to the patient(s).
Homeopathy is generally against artificiality, so a homeopathic doctor will probably recommend the more natural types of contraception (diaphragm, IUD, condoms, etc.).

The birth control pill has a certain number of contraindications (phlebitis, blood clots, varicose veins in the legs, etc.).

This type of contraceptive pill also artificially modifies the biological equilibrium of the body and changes its hormone levels. It should be avoided except for short periods of time. Although the birth control pill doesn't prevent homeopathic drugs from acting, homeopaths generally oppose the pill on principle, and not because it interferes with their treatments.

There is no homeopathic contraceptive.

Contractures

A permanent muscular contraction.

▷ *See* **Muscles.**

Contusions (Bruises)

▷ *See* **Injuries.**

Convalescence

When convalescing from an infectious disease, you may try the following treatment over a two-week period :
SULPHUR IODATUM 9 C,
PULSATILLA 9 C,
TUBERCULINUM AVIARE 9 C,
alternate three pellets of each, three times a day.

Corallium rubrum

Base substance: Red coral.

Characteristic signs and symptoms:
Rapid, repeating cough with purplish facial congestion; abundant mucus in the back of the nose; inhaled air seems cold.

Main clinical uses:
Whooping cough: <u>*WARNING*</u> - *This disease is serious. Contact your physician immediately for treatment recommendation.*
Common cold; spasmodic coughing.

Coryza

▷ *See* **Colds.**

Cosmetic surgery

Plastic surgery consists of reconstructing or reshaping parts of the body. It is a perfectly valid therapeutic practice in certain instances, such as after a disfiguring accident.

"Cosmetic" surgery, on the other hand, is more debatable. Whatever your face or thighs are like, you are a human being and should be respected as such. If you have a complex about your physical appearance, you are suffering from problems inside you as well. If cosmetic surgery is carried out when you're distraught, out-of-step and tired, you run the risk of poor scar healing. A good surgeon will, of course, take the psychological and emotional factors into account.
If you plan on plastic surgery, prepare yourself by looking under the following headings: **Anxiety, Surgery, Scars.**

Coughing

WARNING: When coughing lasts for a long period of time, you must see a doctor.

Yet coughing is a good sign because it eliminates bronchial mucus and germs. But it's also uncomfortable and unpleasant. Coughing can be cured by homeopathic medicines that make a cough disappear when it is no longer useful. Allopathic "cough medicines" stop the cough, but leave purulent mucus inside the bronchial tubes. The homeopathic medicine first reinforces the cough to help it eliminate secretions, then it stops it when the cough no longer plays a useful role.

This method takes longer but is much more beneficial and helps prevent relapses.

Take three pellets of the remedy you have chosen three times a day.

Depending on what started the coughing:
- coughing while swallowing,
  BROMIUM 9 C.
- allergic cough,
  IPECAC 9 C.
- while asleep,
  LACHESIS 9 C.
- set off by touching the larynx,
  LACHESIS 9 C.
- after exertion,
  PULSATILLA 9 C.
- after small drafts of fresh air,
  RUMEX CRISPUS 9 C.
- while speaking or laughing,
  STANNUM METALLICUM 9 C.
- during menstrual periods,
  ZINCUM METALLICUM 9 C.

Depending on circumstances:
Coughing made worse by:
- moving around,
  BRYONIA ALBA 9 C.
- going into an overheated room,
  BRYONIA ALBA 9 C.
- lying down,
  DROSERA ROTUNDIFOLIA 9 C.
- bathing,
  RHUS TOXICODENDRON 9 C.
- going into a cold room,
  RUMEX CRISPUS 9 C.

Coughing made better by:
- burping or passing gas,
  SANGUINARIA CANADENSIS 9 C.
- eating or drinking,
  SPONGIA TOSTA 9 C.

Depending on sensations:
- dry cough,
  BRYONIA ALBA 9 C.
- a sensation that the cough originates in the stomach,
  BRYONIA ALBA 9 C.
- a sensation that the chest is full of mucus because the bronchial passages are paralyzed—no mucus is coughed up,
  CAUSTICUM 9 C.
- nonstop coughing (one coughing fit after another),
  DROSERA ROTUNDIFOLIA 9 C.
- a sensation of irritation and itching of the trachea,
  IPECAC 9 C.
- heavy cough with stringy sputum,
  KALI BICHROMICUM 9 C.
- cough with a sensation of a crumb in the throat,
  LACHESIS 9 C.
- heavy, productive cough during the day; dry cough at night,
  PULSATILLA 9 C.
- hoarse cough that sounds like a dog's bark,
  SPONGIA TOSTA 9 C.

Depending on accompanying symptoms:
- cough with laryngitis, hoarse voice,
  DROSERA ROTUNDIFOLIA 9 C.
- with bleeding of the nose,
  DROSERA ROTUNDIFOLIA 9 C.
- with nausea,
  IPECAC 9 C.
- with suffocation,
  SAMBUCUS NIGRA 9 C.
- with painful vocal cords,
  SPONGIA TOSTA 9 C.

Cracks of the skin

- If the cracks are slightly purulent or yellowish,
   GRAPHITES 9 C,
   three pellets three times a day.
- If the cracks bleed inside,
   NITRICUM ACIDUM 9 C,
   three pellets three times a day.

A local treatment may be necessary. Apply CALENDULA ointment twice a day.
If irritation, bleeding or pain persists, or if infection occurs, consult your doctor.

Cramps

Muscle cramps:
   CUPRUM METALLICUM 9 C,
   NUX VOMICA 9 C,
   alternate three pellets of each, three times a day.
When a cramp occurs, try to stretch the painful muscle: for example, if you get a cramp in your calf, bend your foot back as far as you can, and then gradually pull the toes and the foot toward the front of your leg.

Stomach cramps:
▷ see **Stomach.**

Writer's cramp:
   ARGENTUM NITRICUM 9 C,
   MAGNESIA PHOSPHORICA 9 C,
   alternate three pellets of each, three times a day.

Creosotum

Base substance: Creosote (distillation of Beechwood tar).

Suitable for: Cases of severe irritation of the mucous membranes.

Characteristic signs and symptoms:
Irritating, foul-smelling discharges of the mucous membranes; bleeding of the mucous membranes from the slightest pressure; wedge-shaped, decayed teeth.

Main clinical uses:
Bronchitis; inflammation of the eyelids; gastritis; itching of the vagina; enuresis; decayed teeth.
White vaginal discharge; cervical inflammation: *WARNING - These diseases are serious. You should consult your physician for advice.*

Crocus sativus

Base substance: Saffron.

Characteristic signs and symptoms:
A sensation that something is moving in the abdomen; muscle spasms; varying moods dominated by the need to laugh.

Main clinical use: Fits of hysteria.

Croton tiglium

Base substance: Croton oil.

Characteristic signs and symptoms:
Extremely itchy, vesicular eruptions (scratching is painful), particularly in the genital region; alternation of eruptions and diarrhea.

Main clinical uses:
Eczema or shingles of the genital region: *WARNING - This disease is serious. Contact your physician immediately for treatment recommendation.*

Crowds (Fear of)

Before leaving home, take three pellets of:

ACONITUM NAPELLUS 9 C.
If necessary, renew the dose one hour later.

▷ *Also see* **Agoraphobia.**

Cuprum metallicum

Base substance: Copper.

Characteristic signs and symptoms:
Muscle cramps, violent muscle spasms; hiccups; spasmodic coughing relieved by drinking cold water; diarrhea with crampy pain.

Main clinical uses:
Whooping cough: *WARNING - This disease is serious. Contact your physician immediately for treatment recommendation.*
Intermittent stomach cramps or cramps in legs and soles of feet; spasms; coughs: *WARNING: If condition worsens or persists for more than 72 hours, check with your physician.*

Cure

For homeopathic doctors, illness is a state of imbalance in the body which interferes with the general dynamism (see this entry) of the organism. The word "cure," therefore, indicates a return to an earlier state of equilibrium. A cure is often possible with Homeopathy: symptoms go away and the person feels well again.

Sometimes, Homeopathy can cure diseases of unknown cause. Whenever the pattern of symptoms corresponds to a homeopathic remedy the illness may be curable, no matter what name the disease is given. The doctor obviously prefers to know what ailment he or she is treating but can still prescribe an effective treatment without knowing.

People who have their doubts about Homeopathy can also find a cure for their illnesses with an appropriate homeopathic treatment. In order to choose the right therapy, however, the homeopathic doctor will need the patient's absolute cooperation during the consultation. If the homeopath's questions are not answered with full honesty, it's possible that an erroneous choice of medicine will be made because of it.

Note, a cure in Homeopathy is frequently preceded by a temporary aggravation of symptoms (see **Medicinal aggravation**).

Cuts

▷ *See* **Injuries.**

Cyclamen europaeum

Base substance: Cyclamen.

Characteristic signs and symptoms:
Ophthalmic migraines with the impression of multicolored lights in front of the eyes; "transparent" dizziness—objects are seen as both stationary and mobile at the same time; hiccups during pregnancy; exaggerated scrupulousness.

Main clinical uses:
Ophthalmic migraine, menstrual migraine, sadness.

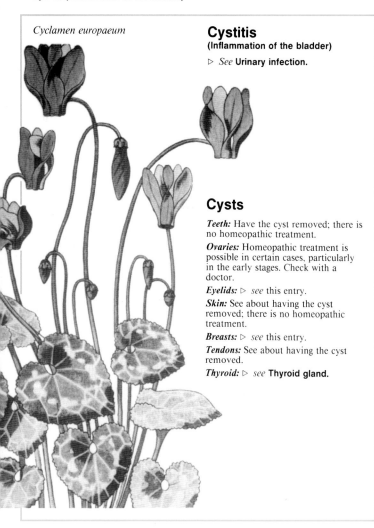

Cyclamen europaeum

Cystitis
(Inflammation of the bladder)

▷ *See* **Urinary infection.**

Cysts

Teeth: Have the cyst removed; there is no homeopathic treatment.

Ovaries: Homeopathic treatment is possible in certain cases, particularly in the early stages. Check with a doctor.

Eyelids: ▷ *see* this entry.

Skin: See about having the cyst removed; there is no homeopathic treatment.

Breasts: ▷ *see* this entry.

Tendons: See about having the cyst removed.

Thyroid: ▷ *see* **Thyroid gland.**

D

*Homeopathy is a
"progressive and aggressive
step in medicine."*

JOHN D. ROCKEFELLER

Dandruff

▷ *See* **Hair.**

Danger in Homeopathy

Homeopathic remedies are generally
viewed as safe medicine. To help you
differentiate between those products
labeled "homeopathic" which are
intended to be potentized by the
manufacturer in preparing
homeopathic drug products and those
homeopathic drug products intended
to be used as the final dosage form,
the normal recommended potencies
for home use have been indicated,
where appropriate.

Low potencies, 4 C and 5 C, are
generally used when symptoms are
first recognized; medium potencies,
7 C and 9 C, are used for general
symptoms; whereas high potencies,
15 C to 30 C, are used for mental and
emotional symptoms.

Do not attempt to use potencies lower
than those recommended, because
some homeopathic products in this
low potency range exist only as base
material or pharmaceutical necessities
and are intended to be used by the
manufacturer to prepare further
homeopathic drug products. Base
materials in some cases may be toxic.
(*See* the **Appendix: Potency Levels.**)
Remember that conditions for which
self-treatment is appropriate usually
fall into the following categories:

• They are self-limiting—that is, they
will resolve themselves in time
without intervention.

• They do not require the immediate
care of a physician.

• They do not require complex
medical diagnosis or monitoring.

You should always remember to
follow recommended dosages and
directions for use, and seek medical
assistance should an acute condition
worsen or persist for more than one to
three days, depending on the particular
illness.

Deafness

Most of the causes for deafness are
organic (see **Organic diseases**) and
Homeopathy cannot help them.
Only anxiety deafness (hearing
decreases during periods of anxiety)
may benefit from:
ARGENTUM NITRICUM 9 C,
three pellets three times a day,
over a period of several months.

Decalcification

▷ *See* **Demineralization, Bones.**

Definition of Homeopathy

▷ *See* **Homeopathic theory.**

Deglutition

▷ *See* **Swallowing.**

Delirium

Homeopathic treatment has little
effect on delirium. Only in rare cases
of delirium can a homeopathic
physician use Homeopathy
exclusively. Nevertheless, if you have
a person around you who is delirious

and you can't reach a doctor, try the following:

- For acute delirium with hallucinations,
    BELLADONNA 9 C,
    three pellets every 15 minutes or every hour.
- For delirium accompanied by quarreling and sexual arousal,
    HYOSCYAMUS NIGER 9 C,
    same dosage.
- For delirium when the patient is highly talkative and shows heightened religious awareness, with wide-open staring eyes,
    STRAMONIUM 9 C,
    same dosage.

Demineralization

Demineralization is a lack of mineral salts, especially of bone and connective tissue. It may be characterized by white spots on the nails.
Take:
    CALCAREA PHOSPHORICA 6 X,
    NATRUM MURIATICUM 6 X,
    two tablets of each of these remedies during the two main meals, twenty days a month for four months.

▷ See **Cell Salts.**

▷ *Note:* The white spots move slowly toward the outer edge of the nail; give them a few months to disappear. Check with your doctor whenever you first notice any bone pain.

Dental caries (Tooth decay)

▷ See **Teeth.**

Dental inflammation

▷ See **Teeth.**

Dentition (Teething)

A tooth coming through: Choose your child's remedy depending on teething symptoms:
- fever,
    ACONITUM NAPELLUS 9 C.
- toothache,
    CHAMOMILLA 9 C.
- a red cheek,
    CHAMOMILLA 9 C.
- diarrhea,
    PODOPHYLLUM PELTATUM 9 C.

Late teething:
    CALCAREA CARBONICA 9 C,
    SILICEA 9 C,
    three pellets of each, three times a day.

▷ See **Homeopathic dentists.**

Deodorant

As for anything that is unnatural, Homeopathy does not advocate deodorants. Often deodorants contain harsh chemicals and drying agents which may interfere with the healthy, normal functioning of the sweat glands by clogging the pores. It's much more logical to wash or shower several times a day if necessary, with pure unscented soap. Proper hygiene is often enough to kill the bacteria that cause perspiration odor.

▷ See **Perspiration.**

Depression

Can Homeopathy alone be effective in cases of mental or emotion distress?

Homeopathy can certainly be effective in the early stages, but so can a lot of love and understanding. You can help relieve distressed people of some of

Mental or emotional distress: at the first sign of sadness, try a homeopathic treatment.

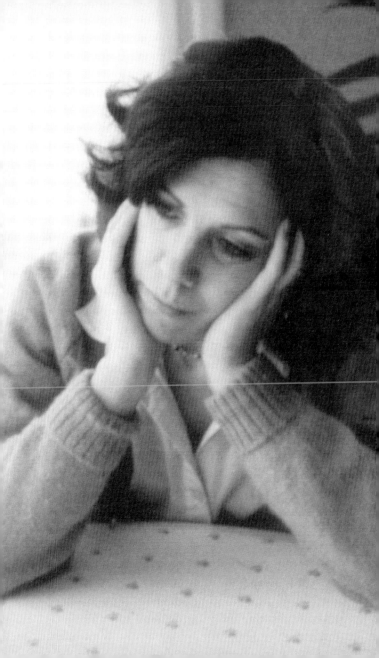

their burdens by talking with them, getting them interested in physical exercise and of course, being sure that they get the proper attention from a homeopathic physician.
Uncontrollable sadness, apathy, loss of self-esteem are some of the warning signs of mental or emotional distress. If they don't improve, absolutely let your doctor know about them. One or more of the following homeopathic remedies (three pellets per day) may be used.

Depending on the cause:
● for depression after being upset, annoyed or bereaved,
   IGNATIA AMARA 9 C.
● from mental strain,
   KALI PHOSPHORICUM 9 C.
● caused by professional problems,
   LYCOPODIUM CLAVATUM 9 C.
● caused by disappointment in love,
   NATRUM MURIATICUM 9 C.
● during menstrual periods or after childbirth,
   SEPIA 9 C.

Depending on the circumstances:
If mental or emotional distress is aggravated by:
● being consoled,
   NATRUM MURIATICUM 9 C.
● music,
   NATRUM SULPHURICUM 9 C.
● being in the dark,
   PHOSPHORUS 9 C.

If improved by:
● eating,
   ANACARDIUM ORIENTALE 9 C.
● being with other people,
   ARSENICUM ALBUM 9 C.

Depending on perceived sensations:
● anxiety and depression at the same time,
   ARSENICUM ALBUM 9 C.
● loss of all hope of being cured ("what's the use of going on with treatment?"),
   ARSENICUM ALBUM 9 C.

● disgust with life,
   AURUM METALLICUM 9 C.
● constant self-reproach, (A doctor must be notified.)
   AURUM METALLICUM 9 C.
● total indifference,
   PHOSPHORICUM ACIDUM 9 C.

Depending on the accompanying symptoms:
● alternating excitation and depression,
   HYOSCYAMUS NIGER 9 C.
● depression accompanied by problems with breathing,
   IGNATIA AMARA 9 C.
● onset of intellectual slowness,
   KALI PHOSPHORICUM 9 C.
● weight loss,
   NATRUM MURIATICUM 9 C.
● tendency to "mull over problems,"
   NATRUM MURIATICUM 9 C.
● thirst,
   NATRUM MURIATICUM 9 C.
● cold sensitivity or intolerance,
   SILICEA 9 C.

Can Homeopathy and Allopathy both treat depression?

This will frequently not be necessary. If Homeopathy is used early enough, it may alone suffice. With certain cases of mental or emotional disturbance, the risk of the patient inflicting self-harm is too great to take any chances: a family doctor or psychiatrist must be aware of the patient's condition. It may be necessary to treat with certain non-homeopathic medicines.
If a regular treatment has already been started and the patient is feeling better, he or she may eventually benefit from seeing a homeopathic doctor. As improvement continues, it may be possible to transfer from one treatment to the other: that is, weaning off the stronger medicines in a gradual fashion and replacing them with homeopathic medicines. Ask advice from your doctor.

Dermatosis, dermatitis

Synonyms for skin disease.

▷ *See* **Skin.**

Desquamation
(Scaling rashes)

Crusted eruptions occurring in various skin disorders.

General treatment:
GRAPHITES 9 C,
MEZEREUM 9 C,
alternate three pellets of each, three times a day until symptoms disappear.

Local treatment:
Apply CALENDULA ointment once or twice a day.

Developmental Delay of Children

WARNING: You should definitely discuss these problems with your physician so that the exact type of delay can be determined. Paying attention to your child's developmental milestones is important—and easy for you to learn!
Depending on the kind of developmental delay, have the child take three pellets of one of the following remedies twenty days a month.

Emotional immaturity:
The child thinks that no one loves him,
PULSATILLA 9 C.

Slow teething:
CALCAREA CARBONICA 9 C.

Walking (delay in):
CALCAREA CARBONICA 9 C.

Mental, intellectual developmental delay:
BARYTA CARBONICA 9 C.

Speaking (delay in):
NATRUM MURIATICUM 9 C.

Weight (delay in reaching normal):
SILICEA 9 C.

School problems; slow learner:
Check with your doctor.

Height (delay in reaching normal):
SILICEA 9 C.

Diabetes

Diabetes is due to an abnormality of the pancreas. It can't be treated with Homeopathy. The best treatment is a strict diet and the classical antidiabetic drugs. This does not, however, exclude Homeopathy from treating the minor disorders that a diabetic patient may suffer from. In some cases, a background homeopathic treatment will allow for the reduction of antidiabetic drugs by restoring a better balance to the person's organism.

Diagnosis

When you consult a homeopathic doctor, he or she will make two diagnoses—one clinical and the other therapeutic.

▷ *See* **Homeopathic consultation.**

Diarrhea

Acute diarrhea may be treated as follows: Take three pellets of the following medications (selected depending on symptoms) three times a day.

<u>*WARNING:*</u> *If there is no immediate improvement, especially with infants and children, discontinue use of the remedies and check with your doctor. Dehydration may result from diarrhea, and this can develop rapidly into a serious health problem.*

Depending on the cause:
- diarrhea occurring after catching a stomach chill,
  ACONITUM NAPELLLUS 9 C.
- after overeating,
  ANTIMONIUM CRUDUM 9 C.
- after eating sugar or candy,
  ARGENTUM NITRICUM 9 C.
- diarrhea of infectious origin,
  ARSENICUM ALBUM 9 C.
- after a haircut,
  BELLADONNA 9 C.
- diarrhea of emotional origin (important event or bad news),
  GELSEMIUM SEMPERVIRENS 9 C.
- diarrhea from eating oysters,
  LYCOPODIUM CLAVATUM 9 C.
- from drinking milk,
  MAGNESIA MURIATICA 9 C.
- after heavy alcohol ingestion,
  NUX VOMICA 9 C.
- after too many laxatives,
  NUX VOMICA 9 C.
- after eating fatty foods,
  PULSATILLA 9 C.
- after eating ice-cream,
  PULSATILLA 9 C.
- after a cold,
  SANGUINARIA CANADENSIS 9 C.
- from eating fruit,
  VERATRUM ALBUM 9 C.
- during menstrual periods,
  VERATRUM ALBUM 9 C.

Depending on circumstances:
- diarrhea is worse after meals, particularly after breakfast,
  NATRUM SULPHURICUM 9 C.
- diarrhea is worse in the early morning and obliges a run from the bed to the bathroom,
  SULPHUR 9 C.

Depending on the appearance of stools:
- semi-solid, semi-liquid stools,
  ANTIMONIUM CRUDUM 9 C.

- watery stools,
  CINCHONA OFFICINALIS 9 C.
- white, colorless stools,
  PHOSPHORICUM ACIDUM 9 C.
- yellowish stools containing bile,
  PODOPHYLLUM PELTATUM 9 C.

Depending on accompanying symptoms:
- the patient is unable to hold back the diarrhea,
  ALOE SOCOTRINA 9 C.
- foul-smelling stools,
  ARSENICUM ALBUM 9 C.
- fatigue after passing stools,
  CINCHONA OFFICINALIS 9 C.
- painless diarrhea,
  CINCHONA OFFICINALIS 9 C.
- painful diarrhea relieved by bending forward,
  COLOCYNTHIS 9 C.
- explosive diarrhea,
  CROTON TIGLIUM 9 C.
- burning stools and bilous vomiting,
  IRIS VERSICOLOR 9 C.
- diarrhea and cold sweats,
  VERATRUM ALBUM 9 C.

Diathesis

The general state that predisposes a person to a particular disease or group of diseases of the same nature, or to metabolic or structural abnormalities.

▷ *See* **Terrain.**

Diet (Restricted)

A restricted or limited diet during illness is usually only necessary to stem acute infectious diseases of the digestive tract (diarrhea). Fever alone usually makes a person weak, so there is no need generally to reduce food intake. Clear liquids and bland, easily digestible foods are recommended instead.

Diet (Therapeutic)

A homeopathic doctor may recommend a specific course of eating and drinking in accordance with the illness being treated and with the long-term treatment undertaken. The clinical symptoms gathered by the doctor give insight into your personality and the possible weak points of terrain. The therapeutic diagnosis enables the selection of a special diet if necessary.

Dietetics

The branch of therapeutics treating of food and drink in relation to health and disease.

▷ See **Diet.**

Difficulty in breathing

If respiratory difficulty is from anxiety, take:
> IGNATIA AMARA 9 C,
> three pellets every hour or three times a day depending on intensity.

WARNING: If condition persists, discontinue use and consult your physician.

▷ See **Shortness of breath.**

Digestion
(Difficulty in digesting, Indigestion)

Here are a few hints that might help if you suffer from upset stomach (dyspepsia) or from indigestion. The following medicines are to be taken three times a day, before or after meals, depending on the symptoms. Take three pellets each time.

For a feeling of heaviness after meals:
- The stomach feels too full and the tongue is coated white,
  > ANTIMONIUM CRUDUM 9 C.
- sensation of a stone in the stomach,
  > BRYONIA ALBA 9 C.
- food takes several hours to be digested,
  > LYCOPODIUM CLAVATUM 9 C.
- person feels bloated after meals,
  > LYCOPODIUM CLAVATUM 9 C.
- the need to take a long nap after meals, then feeling better (a short nap makes things worse),
  > LYCOPODIUM CLAVATUM 9 C.
- the need to take a short nap after meals, then feeling better,
  > NUX VOMICA 9 C.
- the stomach feels much too full and the back of the tongue is coated,
  > NUX VOMICA 9 C.

Before eating a heavy meal that you might not be able to digest, take three pellets of:
> NUX VOMICA 9 C,
> a half hour before the meal starts.

Intolerance to certain foods:
Beer: KALI BICHROMICUM 9 C.
Bread: BRYONIA ALBA 9 C.
Butter: PULSATILLA 9 C.
Cabbage: PETROLEUM 9 C.
Carrots: LYCOPODIUM CLAVATUM 9 C.
Cheese: PTELEA TRIFOLIATA 9 C.
Coffee: IGNATIA AMARA 9 C.
Crawfish: ASTACUS FLUVIATILUS 9 C.
Eggs: FERRUM METALLICUM 9 C.
Fat: PULSATILLA 9 C.
Fish: CHININUM ARSENICOSUM 9 C.
Fruit: CINA 9 C.
Honey: ARGENTUM NITRICUM 9 C.
Ice-cream: PULSATILLA 9 C.
Jam: ARGENTUM NITRICUM 9 C.
Lobster: HOMARUS 9 C.
Meat (all kinds): FERRUM METALLICUM 9 C.
Milk: NITRICUM ACIDUM 9 C.
Onions: LYCOPODIUM CLAVATUM 9 C.
Oysters: LYCOPODIUM CLAVATUM 9 C.
Pastry: PULSATILLA 9 C.

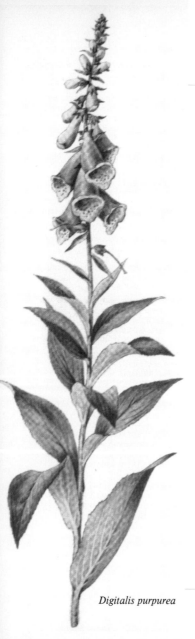

Pork: PULSATILLA 9 C.
Potatoes: ALUMINA 9 C.
Sauerkraut: BRYONIA ALBA 9 C.
Strawberries: FRAGARIA VESCA 9 C.
Sugar: ARGENTUM NITRICUM 9 C.
Tea: SELENIUM 9 C.
Veal: KALI NITRICUM 9 C.
Vegetables: HYDRASTIS
CANADENSIS 9 C.
Wine: NUX VOMICA 9 C.
Vinegar: ANTIMONIUM CRUDUM 9 C.

Person who cannot tolerate the smell of food:
COLCHICUM AUTUMNALE 9 C.

Food poisoning:
ARSENICUM ALBUM 9 C,
PYROGENIUM 9 C,
alternate three pellets of each,
three times a day.

<u>*WARNING:*</u> *Food poisoning is always something to notify your doctor about.*

Hives of dietary origin:
▷ *see* **Urticaria.**

Digitalis purpurea

Base substance: Foxglove.

Characteristic signs and symptoms:
Slow, weak, irregular pulse;
palpitations occurring at the slightest
movement; a sensation as if the heart
were about to stop beating; a need to
be immobile; enlarged liver.

Main clinical uses:
Slow pulse; jaundice in patients with
heart disease: <u>*WARNING*</u> - *These
diseases are serious. Contact your
physician immediately for treatment
recommendation.*

Digitalis purpurea

Dilation of the bronchi

Dilation of the bronchi of the lungs corresponds to damage of the bronchial cartilage. It cannot be treated with Homeopathy. Accompanying infection may benefit from homeopathic treatment.

▷ *See* **Bronchitis.**

Dilution

Dilution is the first step in the process of making homeopathic medicines and one of the most frequently misunderstood aspects of Homeopathy. The *Hahnemannian method* of dilution uses a series of fresh flasks filled with diluent. A certain amount of the mother tincture (or the preceding potency) is added to each flask. Then, between each series of dilution, the flasks undergo another important homeopathic procedure, **potentization,** (see this entry) or vigorous shaking. The remedy is thus diluted and shaken successively, using the previous potency each time, until the desired dilution strength is reached.

The *Korsakov contact method* uses a single vial which is emptied at each potency. The amount of preceding potency left clinging to the vial is all that is mixed with the diluent to form the new potency. Knowing the size of the vial and the surface tension of the liquid allows the calculation of the amount of residual liquid left in the vial and consequent adjustment of the amount of diluent.
Centesimal scale dilutions are those prepared by adding 1 ml of remedy to 99 ml of diluent at each successive step. Thus, a 6 C Hahnemannian potency is prepared by diluting 1 ml of remedy in 99 ml of diluent six times. A 6 K potency is prepared using the same degree of dilution according to the Korsakov contact method.
The same procedures are used for the *decimal scale,* with the exception that dilution is carried out at a ratio of one to ten (1 part medicine to 9 parts diluent). These potencies are designated by the letter 'X', for example, a 1 X, 2 X, 3 X potency, etc. Below is a chart which may help to clear up some confusion:
(*'Designation'* refers to the potency on the label of your remedy; *'scale'* is the amount of dilution at each successive step; and *'method'* refers to the way in which dilution is manufactured.)

Designation	Scale	Method	Synonyms
X	Decimal (1:10)	Hahnemannian	D
D	Decimal (1:10)	Hahnemannian	X
C	Centesimal (1:100)	Hahnemannian	CH
CH	Centesimal (1:100)	Hahnemannian	C
K	Centesimal (1:100)	Korsakov	-
CK	Centesimal (1:100)	Korsakov	K
LM	Fifty Millesimal		-

▷ *See* **Homeopathic theory.**

Dioscorea villosa

Base substance: the Wild yam.

Characteristic signs and symptoms:
Cramp-like pains in the abdomen which are relieved by straightening up or leaning back; pain in the fingers and ears.

Main clinical uses:
Cramps or colic (abdominal, hepatic, renal); whitlow (or felon: a purulent infection on the tip of a finger): _WARNING - These diseases are serious. Contact your physician immediately for treatment recommendation._
Sciatica.

Diseases

How do homeopathic physicians define disease?

A disease is a state of imbalance in the body that interferes with the body's vitality. This disequilibrium is usually caused by outside aggressions (environment, germs, food problems, trauma, psychological problems).
For the homeopathic physician, the disease itself is not the only important thing: the individual and his or her characteristic symptoms (see **Symptom**) are of greater importance, for these alone will enable a homeopathic doctor to select the appropriate treatment for each person's needs.

Acute diseases, chronic diseases

Acute, short-term diseases may be rapidly cured with Homeopathy. If the disease (asthma, for example) recurs several times despite medication, the **terrain** (see this entry) needs treatment. The homeopathic physician

may then question whether the patient is suffering from a chronic disease, and take into account not only acute symptoms but also chronic problems occurring between attacks.

What kind of diseases can most effectively be treated with Homeopathy?

The main types of diseases that Homeopathy is appropriate for are:
• **functional disease** (see this entry),
• **allergies** (see this entry),
• benign infectious diseases,
• skin diseases,
• nervous diseases (anxiety, insomnia, depression),
• digestive problems (hepatic insufficiency, gastroenteritis, gastritis, hepatitis, gastro-duodenal ulcers),
• migraines,
• certain gynecological problems (for example, menstrual cramps and premenstrual syndrome—PMS),
• childhood diseases (see **Children**).
• rheumatism, pain (the cause of the pain cannot always be changed).

Distress (Aftereffects of)

▷ _See_ **Cause of Illnesses, Depression, Emotion.**

Dolichos pruriens

Base substance: Cowage.

Characteristic signs and symptoms:
Itching of the skin without rash or outbreak; sallow skin.

Main clinical uses:
Itching without apparent cause; itching in the elderly.
Itching due to jaundice: _WARNING - This disease is serious. You should consult your physician for advice._

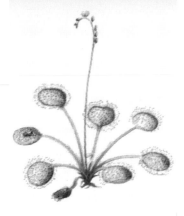

Dosage

Understanding the general principles of dosage in Homeopathy assumes that you're familiar with the ideas of similarity and infinitesimal (see **Homeopathic theory**).

The closer the similarity between a person's symptoms and the experimental symptoms inherent to the action of the remedy being prescribed, the greater the possibility of using a high potency successfully. Homeopaths generally recommend a medium potency preparation of a homeopathic medicine (in most cases, the 9 C, or the 9th Hahnemannian centesimal). *The Guide* follows this recommendation. Three pellets (from a multi-dose tube) are traditionally prescribed for all ages: the dose is the same for children, adults and elderly people.

A unit-dose tube is a small tube containing tiny medicated granules (pellets size 20). Its entire contents should be taken at once and should only be taken again after your doctor has given the go-ahead.

▷ *See* **Homeopathic medicines, Prescriptions.**

Down's syndrome
(Trisomy 21)

Unfortunately, Down's syndrome cannot be cured with any medicine since it is a congenital, chromosomal abnormality (trisomy 21).

Drosera rotundifolia

Base substance: the Sundew plant.
Characteristic signs and symptoms:
Barking, paroxysmal cough with

sensation of inspiratory suffocation; tickling in the larynx, hoarseness, nosebleeds and stridor (a high-pitched breathing sound, like a cock's crow, that comes from airway obstruction); chest pain and abdominal pain when coughing; coughing aggravated by alcohol; coughing aggravated by lying down.

Main clinical uses:
Coughing; asthma.
Whooping cough; laryngitis:
<u>*WARNING*</u> - *These diseases are serious. Contact your physician immediately for treatment recommendation.*

Drowsiness

For drowsiness after meals, take three pellets of the following before the two main meals:
• if drowsiness is improved by a short nap,
NUX VOMICA 9 C.
• if drowsiness is worsened by a nap,
LYCOPODIUM CLAVATUM 9 C.

Dulcamara

Base substance: Bittersweet.
Suitable for: People who are sensitive to wet weather.

Characteristic signs and symptoms:
Rheumatic pains when the weather is humid; urticaria (hives) before menstrual periods; wide, flat, smooth warts; diarrhea in warm weather.

Main clinical uses:
Rheumatism; inflammation of the mucous membranes; warts; facial neuralgia (tics); diarrhea.

Duodenum

Duodenal ulcers should be treated like stomach ulcers.

▷ *See* **Stomach.**

Dupuytren's contracture

This condition is a retraction and hardening of the flexor tendons of the palms, leading to sustained flexion of the fingers. Once the disease has set in and become a hindrance, surgery may be the only solution.

Dynamism

Homeopathic medicines obviously do not act because of the quantity of medicine in them, as this is infinitesimal (see **Homeopathic theory**). The only way to explain their action is to admit that these medicines have a dynamic strength or force. By their energy, they probably furnish a kind of coded signal that tells the body to react in a certain way. According to this concept, restoring a proper dynamic equilibrium to the organism brings back good health; in other words, the medicines reestablish a proper balance between the things on the outside that might attack the body and the body's own self-defenses against disease. This concept is indispensable to a full understanding of Homeopathy. What it comes down to is that the modern expression of the old idea of "vital energy" corresponds to reality, a reality which can certainly be experienced by each person, even if it has yet to be conclusively proven.

▷ *See* **Reactional Mode.**

Dysentery

Don't try to diagnose dysentery yourself. Your physician should be the one to run tests to see whether or not you have this disease. An appropriate homeopathic treatment can then be prescribed.

▷ *See* **Diarrhea.**

Dyshidrosis

▷ *See* **Eczema.**

Dysmenorrhea

Painful menstruation.

▷ *See* **Menstrual periods.**

Dyspepsia

Poor digestion.

▷ *See* **Digestion.**

Dyspnea

▷ *See* **Difficulty in breathing, Shortness of breath.**

Dysuria (Strangury)

Difficulty in urinating.

▷ *See* **Urinating.**

EFG

*"An enormous mass of experience,
both of homeopathic doctors
and their patients,
is invoked in favor of the efficacy
of these remedies and doses."*

WILLIAM JAMES
(American philosopher & psychologist, 1842-1910)

Ears

▷ *See* **Ringing in the ears, Mastoiditis, Otitis.**

Ecchymosis (Bruises)

▷ *See* **Injuries.**

Ecology

Homeopathy is the safe, natural, and ecological healing art "par excellence" because it respects the laws of human nature.
Unlike **Allopathy** (see this entry), which fights disease with drugs producing an aggressive reaction inside the body, Homeopathy heals by remedies that incite the body to rid itself of the illness.

Eczema

Homeopathy can act in quite a very positive way in this illness. Choose one or two of the following remedies, depending on the outbreak or rash, and take three pellets three times a day of each.

Depending on the cause:
- eczema in a big eater,
  ANTIMONIUM CRUDUM 9 C.
- eczema after a vaccination,
  MEZEREUM 9 C.

Depending on modifying circumstances:
Eczema aggravated by:
- seawater,
  NATRUM MURIATICUM 9 C.
- the sun,
  NATRUM MURIATICUM 9 C.
- winter weather,
  PETROLEUM 9 C.
- water,
  SULPHUR 9 C.

- the heat,
  SULPHUR 9 C.

Improved by:
- the heat,
  ARSENICUM ALBUM 9 C.
- the cold,
  SULPHUR 9 C.

Depending on the appearance of the rash:
- pink-colored eczema,
  APIS MELLIFICA 9 C.
- dry eczema like a fine powder,
  ARSENICUM ALBUM 9 C.
- dry, scaly eczema,
  ARSENICUM IODATUM 9 C.
- with red skin,
  BELLADONNA 9 C.
- with large blisters,
  CANTHARIS 9 C.
- with oozing,
  GRAPHITES 9 C.
- with scabs,
  MEZEREUM 9 C.
- with bleeding cracks,
  NITRICUM ACIDUM 9 C.
- with blisters,
  RHUS TOXICODENDRON 9 C.
- in case of dyshidrosis (small, clear blisters on the hands and feet),
  RHUS VENENATA 9 C.

Depending on the location:
- anus,
  BERBERIS VULGARIS 9 C.
- mouth (around the mouth),
  SEPIA 9 C.
- scalp,
  OLEANDER 9 C.
- elbow (inside the bend of the arm),
  BERBERIS VULGARIS 9 C.
- forehead,
  NATRUM MURIATICUM 9 C.
- knees (behind the knee),
  CEREUS BOMPLANDII 9 C.
- hand (back of),
  PIX LIQUIDA 9 C.
- palm,
  ANAGALLIS 9 C.
- finger tips,
  PETROLEUM 9 C.
- ears (behind the ears),
  GRAPHITES 9 C.

• in the external auditory canal of the ear,
    PSORINUM 9 C.
• genital region,
    CROTON TIGLIUM 9 C.
• foot: horny, calloused eczema,
    ANTIMONIUM CRUDUM 9 C.
• foot: cracked eczema,
    LYCOPODIUM CLAVATUM 9 C.
Be sure to check with a homeopathic physician if you suffer from chronic eczema.

Edema

An accumulation of an excessive amount of fluid causing swelling of the tissues, particularly of the subcutaneous connective tissues, due largely to problems of circulatory origin. Most causes are organic, so check with your doctor.

Elbow pains

▷ *See* **Rheumatism.**

After choosing a treatment from the list under Rheumatism, supplement it with the following:
    RHUS TOXICODENDRON 9 C,
    three pellets three times a day.

▷ *Also see* **Epicondylitis.**

Embolism

No matter where it occurs in the body, embolism (obstruction of an artery or vein by a clot of blood, an air bubble, etc.), is not within the realm of homeopathic treatment. Regular medical treatment is absolutely necessary. Homeopathy, however, can treat some of the physical consequences of emboli. Consult your doctor.

Emergencies in Homeopathy

Homeopathy may be quite effective in some cases of emergency. It's often mistakenly thought that Homeopathy always works slowly and only works in chronic diseases. Homeopathic medicines can have a truly spectacular effect in treating some acute diseases.

▷ *See* the appropriate sections for further information.

Emotion (Consequences of)

Depending on the cause, take three pellets three times a day of one of the following medicines:
• after fear,
    ACONITUM NAPELLUS 9 C.
• for apprehension prior to an event,
    ARGENTUM NITRICUM 9 C.
• for upset from anger,
    COLOCYNTHIS 9 C.
• after bad news,
    GELSEMIUM SEMPERVIRENS 9 C.
• following setback, grief or bereavement,
    IGNATIA AMARA 9 C.
• for intellectual overwork,
    KALI PHOSPHORICUM 9 C.
• for unrequited love,
    NATRUM MURIATICUM 9 C.
• after irritation or annoyance,
    STAPHYSAGRIA 9 C.

▷ *Also consult* the appropriate sections regarding your symptoms, particularly **Anxiety.**

Emphysema

Emphysema (dilation and destruction of the alveoli, or air spaces, of the lung, often from smoking) cannot be cured by Homeopathy. **Asthma** and certain types of **bronchitis,** on the other hand, may respond to homeopathic treatment.

Empiricism

▷ *See* **Philosophy.**

Encephalitis (Aftereffects of)

Encephalitis has several causes, most of which are viral. The disease varies in severity, and very mild cases may benefit from some homeopathic treatments.

WARNING: Always consult a physician first whenever you or a child suffer from fever and a sore neck or mental confusion.

For the aftereffects of a former case of encephalitis, try three pellets of:
> HELLEBORUS NIGER 9 C,
> three times a day, twenty days a month for a few months.

Enteritis
(Intestinal inflammation)

▷ *See* **Diarrhea.**

It is not within the scope of this guide to discuss the difference between enteritis and the other causes of diarrhea. Suffice it to say, the symptomatic treatment is the same. Diagnosis should be made by your physician.

Enuresis (Bed-wetting)

Toilet-trained children who wet the bed at night are suffering from an illness, one as real as any other illness: enuresis.
Above all, parents should be careful not to overdramatize the situation. Don't scold the child when an "accident" occurs, and don't offer praise when the bed stays dry overnight. Avoid using any kind of device on children designed to shock or wake them when urinating in bed. Remember, your child is just as embarrassed about the situation as you are. A homeopathic doctor can help; the treatment will take about a year. But you can start with these remedies while waiting to see the doctor.
● for restless sleep, when the child talks in his or her sleep, and dreams about urinating,
> BELLADONNA 9 C,
> three pellets three times a day.
● if the urine has a strong smell,
> BENZOICUM ACIDUM 9 C,
> taken as above.
● for enuresis alone, without any other particular symptoms,
> EQUISETUM HYEMALE 6 X,
> three pellets three times a day.
● if the child spoils the bed (defecates) and urinates at the same time,
> HYOSCYAMUS NIGER 9 C,
> taken as above.
● if the child urinates only early in the night,
> SEPIA 9 C,
> taken as above.

Epicondylitis

Epicondylitis or "tennis elbow" (pain on the outside of the elbow joint) isn't something that all tennis players suffer from. Those that do should take a close look at their playing technique. Anyone, however, suffering from "tennis elbow" should take:
> RHUS TOXICODENDRON 9 C,
> three pellets three times a day until improvement.
Apply locally RUTA GRAVEOLENS M.T.: twenty-five drops on a compress three times a day.

Epididymitis

WARNING: Check with your doctor.
Inflammation of the epididymis, the

first portion of the excretory duct of the testis. Take:

> PULSATILLA 9 C,
> RHODODENDRON
> CHRYSANTHEMUM 9 C,
> SPONGIA TOSTA 9 C,
> alternate three pellets of each, three times a day.

Epilepsy

Epilepsy is not curable by Homeopathy. Homeopathic medicines can only help the classical medications prescribed for this illness. Homeopathy can also help to calm the epileptic patient's anxiety. See your homeopathic doctor.

Epistaxis

Nosebleed.

▷ *See* **Bleeding.**

Equilibrium

▷ *See* **Gait.**

Erection (Difficulty in attaining)

▷ *See* **Sexual disorders.**

Eructation, aerophagy, belching

Take one or more of the following medicines (three pellets three times a day) depending on the circumstances:
• for frequent belching,
> ARGENTUM NITRICUM 9 C.
• for loud belching,
> ARGENTUM NITRICUM 9 C.
• for belching after being annoyed about something,
> ARGENTUM NITRICUM 9 C.

• for belching that leaves a "rotten egg" taste in the mouth,
> ARNICA MONTANA 9 C.
• if the air moves slowly up the esophagus, like a rising ball,
> ASAFOETIDA 9 C.
• for belching that relieves bloatedness,
> CARBO VEGETABILIS 9 C.
• for belching that leaves an aftertaste of food,
> CARBO VEGETABILIS 9 C.
• for belching from overeating,
> CARBO VEGETABILIS 9 C.
• for belching that does not relieve bloatedness,
> CINCHONA OFFICINALIS 9 C.
• for belching caused by eating bread,
> HYDRASTIS CANADENSIS 9 C.

Erysipelas

This inflammatory skin disease can be serious because of the fever and severe physical symptoms which accompany it. Painful red skin and blisters, which are caused by streptococcus bacteria, are signs of this disease. It is absolutely essential to consult a physician. Homeopathy may be effective.

Erythema nodosum

The formation of painful red nodes of rheumatic (streptococcal) or drug-sensitivity origin on the legs. This rash may be treated by Homeopathy. Check with your physician.

Esophagus

For problems of the esophagus, take three pellets of one of the following remedies before every meal:
• the sensation of a rising lump in the esophagus,
> ASAFOETIDA 9 C.

- burning pains in the esophagus during a migraine headache,
  IRIS VERSICOLOR 9 C.
- burning sensations inside the esophagus after meals,
  NUX VOMICA 9 C.

▷ If you suffer from spasms of the esophagus (food becomes stuck behind the sternum after swallowing), check with your doctor.

Etymology of the term "Homeopathy"

▷ See **History of Homeopathy**.

Eugenia jambos

Base substance: the seeds of the Malabar plum tree.

Characteristic signs and symptoms: Juvenile acne in the form of indurated, painful pimples.

Main clinical use: Juvenile acne.

Eupatorium perfoliatum

Base substance: Ague weed, also known as Boneset.

Characteristic signs and symptoms: Fever with a sensation that the bones are breaking; thirst followed by shivering; fever without perspiration; bilious vomiting during bouts of fever; pain in the eyeballs.

Main clinical uses: Flu-like symptoms, particularly with aching pain and stiffness, fever, restlessness, intense thirst.

WARNING: If condition worsens or persists for more than 72 hours, check with your physician.

Euphrasia officinalis

Base substance: Eyebright.

Characteristic signs and symptoms: Eye inflammation with abundant watering that burns the lower eyelid; sensitivity to light; blinking of the eyes; inflammation of the nose and non-irritating discharge.

Main clinical uses: Conjunctivitis; coryza; hay fever.

WARNING: If condition worsens or persists for more than 72 hours, check with your physician.

Examinations (Preparing for)

▷ See **Nervousness before an Event**.

Exhibitionism

▷ See **Sexual Disorders**.

Experimentation

Experimentation of medicines in the discipline of Homeopathy is carried out on human beings. People in apparently good health are given subtoxic doses of the experimental medicines. All the symptoms observed in the experimental subjects from a given substance are noted, and their compilation represents what is known as the "pathogenesis" or "proving" of the remedy. With this knowledge, a physician may later apply the Law of Similars (see **Homeopathic theory**) and choose a homeopathic medicine that causes the same symptom picture, or group of symptoms. The experimental basis of Homeopathy makes it a reliable and scientific branch of medicine.

For fundamental scientific research in Homeopathy, ▷ *see* **Research (Scientific - in Homeopathy).**

Eyebrows (Falling out of)

Take:
> FLUORICUM ACIDUM 9 C,
> three pellets three times a day, two weeks a month over a period of several months.

Eyelashes (Falling out of)

Take:
> FLUORICUM ACIDUM 5 C,
> three pellets three times a day, ten days a month over a period of several months.

Eyelids

Chalazion:
This small cyst, or granuloma, of the eyelids may sometimes have to be removed or lanced by an eye doctor. If so, take the following remedies to avoid relapses:
> STAPHYSAGRIA 9 C,
> THUJA OCCIDENTALIS 9 C,
> alternate three pellets of each, three times a day over a period of three months.

Eyelids that stick together in the morning:
> GRAPHITES 9 C,
> three pellets three times a day.

Inflamed eyelids (blepharitis):
> GRAPHITES 9 C,
> same dosage.

WARNING: If condition worsens or persists for more than 72 hours, check with your physician.

Cysts (Inflammation of):
▷ *see* **Styes.**

Ptosis (Drooping of the eyelids):
> CAUSTICUM 9 C,
> three pellets three times a day.

Spasms:
> BELLADONNA 9 C,
> three pellets three times a day.

Eyes

Good vision is priceless.

WARNING: Check with an eye doctor whenever you or your family have the slightest worry about an infection, injury or change of vision.

Cataract:
Homeopathy can't make cataracts regress, but it can help slow down their evolution.

Conjunctivitis:
The conjunctiva is the delicate membrane covering the front of each eye. Your doctor should know whenever you have any inflammation of your conjunctivae.
General treatment (three pellets of the chosen remedy three times daily):
- conjunctivitis after a dry chill to the eye,
> ACONITUM NAPELLUS 9 C.
- with non-irritating watering of the eyes,
> ALLIUM CEPA 9 C.
- if the conjunctivae are swollen (a raised area around the iris),
> APIS MELLIFICA 9 C.
- dark red conjunctivae,
> BELLADONNA 9 C.
- light red conjunctivae,
> EUPHRASIA OFFICINALIS 9 C.
- with watering that irritates the lower eyelid,
> EUPHRASIA OFFICINALIS 9 C.
- with irritating pus (Notify your doctor of any pus.),
> MERCURIUS CORROSIVUS 9 C.
- with non-irritating pus (Notify your doctor.),
> PULSATILLA 9 C.

Glaucoma: ▷ *see* this entry. (You must see an eye doctor.)

"Floaters" before the eyes (this is frequently due to harmless, natural residue inside the liquid of the eye, and without serious consequences):
PHOSPHORUS 9 C,
three pellets three times a day whenever bothersome.

Strabismus (squint): ▷ *see* this entry.

Styes: ▷ *see* this entry.

Trauma of the eye:
You must be examined immediately by an eye doctor.

If you have been hit in the eye, resulting in bruising of the soft area around the eye:
LEDUM PALUSTRE 9 C,
three pellets three times a day.

If you have been hit in the eyeball, but with no bruising:
SYMPHYTUM OFFICINALE 9 C,
same dosage as above.

Eyesight disorders: ▷ *see* below, **Eyesight.**

Eyesight

Nearsightedness, farsightedness, presbyopia and astigmatism are not within the range of Homeopathy.

Tiredness of the eyes may be avoided by taking:
RUTA GRAVEOLENS 30 C,
one unit-dose tube per week.

Face

For cases of sudden, violent pains in the face (facial neuralgia), take three pellets of one of the following remedies three to ten times a day:
• facial neuralgia from exposure to dry cold,
   ACONITUM NAPELLUS 9 C.
• relieved by hot compresses,
   ARSENICUM ALBUM 9 C.
• very violent pain,
   BELLADONNA 9 C.
• red, hot face,
   BELLADONNA 9 C.
• relieved by cold compresses,
   COFFEA CRUDA 9 C.
• aggravated by noise,
   SPIGELIA 9 C.

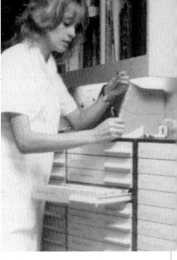

Making up a prescription

False croup

▷ *See* **Laryngitis.**

Family doctor

▷ *See* **the Homeopathic physician.**

Family kit

To treat everyday ailments, it is a good idea to keep the following thirty-five remedies on hand, either in your family medicine cabinet or in a self-care kit to use when traveling.

ACONITUM NAPELLUS 9 C,
ANTIMONIUM CRUDUM 9 C,
ANTIMONIUM TARTARICUM 9 C,
APIS MELLIFICA 9 C,
ARGENTUM NITRICUM 9 C,
ARNICA MONTANA 9 C,
ARSENICUM ALBUM 9 C,
BELLADONNA 9 C,
BRYONIA ALBA 9 C,
CARBO VEGETABILIS 9 C,
CHAMOMILLA 9 C,
CINA 9 C,
CINCHONA OFFICINALIS 9 C,
COFFEA CRUDA 9 C,
COLOCYNTHIS 9 C,
EUPATORIUM PERFOLIATUM 9 C,
EUPHRASIA OFFICINALIS 9 C,
GELSEMIUM SEMPERVIRENS 9 C,

HEPAR SULPHURIS CALCAREUM 9 C,
IGNATIA AMARA 9 C,
IPECACUANHA 9 C,
LACHESIS 9 C,
LYCOPODIUM CLAVATUM 9 C,
MAGNESIA PHOSPHORICA 9 C,
MERCURIUS SOLUBILIS 9 C,
NUX VOMICA 9 C,
PHOSPHORICUM ACIDUM 9 C,
PHOSPHORUS 9 C,
PODOPHYLLUM PELTATUM 9 C,
PULSATILLA 9 C,
RHUS TOXICODENDRON 9 C,
RUTA GRAVEOLENS 9 C,
SAMBUCUS NIGRA 9 C,
SILICEA 9 C,
SULPHUR 9 C.

Fatigue

Fatigue is a *positive symptom*. It sends a warning to the body that it is in need of energy. Don't ignore this message. As much as possible, cut down on your activities and allow enough time for sleeping and eating correctly.

Check with a doctor should you continue to feel tired.

Fortifiers:

Fortifiers, or stimulants as such, do not exist in Homeopathy. A standard homeopathic remedy if properly chosen according to the person's symptoms will act better than the best tonic.

Nonetheless, if you're not ill but you feel the need for a temporary "lift," take three pellets of one of the following remedies three times a day:

• for tiredness resulting from physical strain or trauma,
  ARNICA MONTANA 9 C.
• for fatigue resulting from rapid growth spurt,
  CALCAREA PHOSPHORICA 9 C.
• for fatigue from the loss of a large amount of body fluid (diarrhea, heavy menstrual periods, heavy sweating, vomiting),
  CINCHONA OFFICINALIS 9 C.
• for fatigue from staying up late, or from insomnia,
  COCCULUS INDICUS 9 C.
• for fatigue after hearing bad news,
  GELSEMIUM SEMPERVIRENS 9 C.
• for fatigue and thinness despite a healthy appetite,
  IODIUM 9 C.
• for psychic fatigue,
  KALI PHOSPHORICUM 9 C.
• for convalescing from an infectious disease,
  PULSATILLA 9 C.
• for stiffness after sports,
  RHUS TOXICODENDRON 9 C.
• for fatigue after childbirth,
  SEPIA 9 C.

Fear

A moderate amount of fear is normal; it helps us to protect ourselves and our families from life's dangers. When fear gets to the point that it dominates our lives, however, it is pathological and should be treated.

Try one of the following remedies (three pellets three times a day, twenty days a month over a period of several months):

Fear of animals:
  BELLADONNA 9 C.

Fear of the future:
  CALCAREA CARBONICA 9 C.

Claustrophobia (fear of enclosed places):
  ARGENTUM NITRICUM 9 C,

Fear of going insane:
  CIMICIFUGA RACEMOSA 9 C.

Fear of crowds:
  ACONITUM NAPELLUS 9 C.

Fear of heights:
  ARGENTUM NITRICUM 9 C.

Fear of becoming ill:
  PHOSPHORUS 9 C.

Fear of death:
  ACONITUM NAPELLUS 9 C.

Fear of the dark:
  STRAMONIUM 9 C.

Fear of storms:
  PHOSPHORUS 9 C.

Fear of being inside tunnels:
  STRAMONIUM 9 C.

Fear of robbers:
  NATRUM MURIATICUM 9 C.

▷ *Also see* **Emotion** (for the aftereffects of fear).

Feet

▷ *See* **Bunions, Rheumatism.**

Ferrum metallicum

Base substance: Iron.

Suitable for: People with anemia.

Characteristic signs and symptoms:
Anemia with paleness of the skin and the mucous membranes, and congestion of the circulation; a tendency to bleed; painless diarrhea; rheumatism of the shoulders, improved by slow movement.

Main clinical uses:
Anemia, bleeding:
WARNING - These conditions are serious. Contact your physician immediately for treatment recommendation.
Rheumatism of the shoulder.

Ferrum phosphoricum

Base substance: Ferroso-Ferric Phosphate.

Characteristic signs and symptoms:
Moderately high fever with the color of the face turning alternately pale and red; nosebleeds during fever attacks; rheumatic pains during fever attacks; incontinence of urine; inflammation of the ears and lungs; diarrhea.

Main clinical uses:
Otitis: *WARNING - This disease is serious. Contact your physician immediately for treatment recommendation.*
Early stages of a febrile illness; a tendency to nosebleeds; bronchitis; pulmonary congestion; viral pneumonia; fever with sudden respiratory congestion: *WARNING: If condition worsens or persists for more than 72 hours, check with your physician.*

Fever

Fever is a *positive sign.* Its presence indicates that the body is fighting off an infectious agent (bacteria, virus or parasite). Fever's job is to eliminate the intruder, or to at least prevent it from spreading. It is best, therefore, not to immediately break a fever with antipyretics or mask it with antibiotics unless there is a clear-cut problem or complication.

If the fever is mild—under 39°C or 100°F—you may wish to treat it yourself with the medicines below. Take three pellets of one or more of the following remedies, three times a day (depending on symptoms):

Depending on the cause:
- for fever during cold, dry weather,
  ACONITUM NAPELLUS 9 C.
- for fever from exposure to the cold during a period of hot, dry weather,
  ACONITUM NAPELLUS 9 C.
- for fever during wet weather,
  DULCAMARA 9 C.
- following a cold bath,
  RHUS TOXICODENDRON 9 C.

Depending on the accompanying symptoms:
- for fever with worry, restlessness and fear of death,
  ACONITUM NAPELLUS 9 C.
- with dizziness and paleness when sitting up in bed,
  ACONITUM NAPELLUS 9 C.
- fever with sweating,
  ACONITUM NAPELLUS 9 C.
- fever without sweating,
  BELLADONNA 9 C.
- with red, hot cheeks,
  BELLADONNA 9 C.
- with dilated pupils,
  BELLADONNA 9 C.
- with sleepwalking, convulsions or muttering (on the limit of delirium),
  BELLADONNA 9 C.

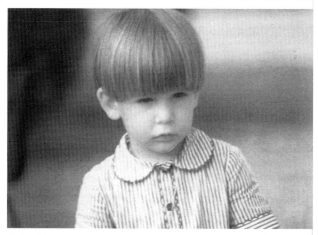

A feverish child may feel faint or unsteady. If symptoms persist, consult your doctor.

- when a person doesn't want to move,
  BRYONIA ALBA 9 C.
- with flushed cheeks or nosebleeds,
  FERRUM PHOSPHORICUM 9 C.
- a feeling of heaviness or lethargy,
  GELSEMIUM SEMPERVIRENS 9 C.
- sensitivity to the cold,
  NUX VOMICA 9 C.
- muscular pain,
  PYROGENIUM 9 C.
- the need to move the muscles,
  RHUS TOXICODENDRON 9 C.

WARNING: If symptoms persist, discontinue use of the above remedies and consult your physician.

▷ Fever is only a sign, not a diagnosis. If other signs and symptoms characteristic of a particular disease seem to be apparent, you should check other headings in this book.

Fever blisters

▷ *See* **Herpes.**

Fifth disease
(Erythema infectiosum)

This is a benign childhood disease of unknown cause which brings on a red rash. Give:
  PULSATILLA 9 C,
  three pellets three times a day over a period of five or six days.

Fingers

Cramps in the fingers:
MAGNESIA PHOSPHORICA 9 C,
three pellets three times a day.

Deformed, knotted, ankylosed fingers:
KALI IODATUM 9 C,
three pellets three times a day,
two weeks per month over a
period of several months.

Squashed or smashed fingers:
ARNICA MONTANA 9 C,
HYPERICUM PERFORATUM 9 C,
alternate three pellets of each, once
an hour or three times a day,
depending on intensity of pain.

Frostbite: ▷ *see* this entry.

Cracking: ▷ *see* **Cracks of the skin,
Eczema.**

Loss of feeling in the fingers:
SECALE CORNUTUM 5 C,
three pellets three times a day.

Rheumatism:
KALI IODATUM 9 C,
three pellets three times a day.
Also be sure to follow one of the
treatments indicated under the
heading, **Rheumatism.**

First aid kit

▷ *See* **Family kit.**

Fissures

▷ *See* **Anus, Eczema.**

Fistula

▷ *See* **Anus, Teeth.**

Flatulence, Gas

▷ *See* **Bloatedness, Eructation.**

For problems of passing gas, take three
pellets of one of the following
remedies three times a day:
- if the gas burns, or feels hot,
ALOE SOCOTRINA 9 C.
- if the gas occurs with diarrhea,
ALOE SOCOTRINA 9 C.
- if the gas smells fetid ,
ARSENICUM ALBUM 9 C.
- if the gas feels cold,
CONIUM MACULATUM 9 C.
- if the gas is difficult to pass,
LYCOPODIUM CLAVATUM 9 C.
- if passing gas relieves the feeling of
bloatedness,
LYCOPODIUM CLAVATUM 9 C.
- if gas seems to be stuck under the
heart,
MOMORDICA BALSAMINA 9 C.

Flea bites

Take:
PULEX IRRITANS 5 C,
three pellets three times a day for
three days.

Flu-like symptoms

▷ *See* **Influenza.**

Fluoricum acidum

Base substance: Fluorhydric acid.

Suitable for:
Elderly, euphoric people who are
indifferent to those around them.

Characteristic signs and symptoms:
Fistulae (around the anus, tear ducts
or mouth); bone necrosis; ulceration of
the skin and mucous membranes;
varicose veins; itchy scars and orifices;
brittle nails and hair.

Main clinical uses: Fistulae, ulcers, bone necrosis.

Formica rufa

Base substance: the Red ant.

Characteristic signs and symptoms: Attacks of gout with profuse sweating; urine full of urates.

Main clinical uses: Gout, cystitis: <u>WARNING</u> - These diseases are serious. Contact your physician immediately for treatment recommendation.

Fractures

To help a bone fracture heal, take the following remedies until you have the cast removed:
SYMPHYTUM OFFICINALE 9 C, three pellets three times a day and CALCAREA PHOSPHORICA 6 X, two tablets three times a day.

Fraxinus americana

Base substance: The American ash tree.

Characteristic signs and symptoms: Uterine fibroma with a sensation of heaviness in the lower pelvic region; vaginal discharge; prolapse of organs.

Main clinical uses: Fibroma, prolapse of organs: <u>WARNING</u> - These diseases are extremely serious. Contact your physician immediately for treatment recommendation.

Fright (Consequences of)

▷ *See* **Emotion.**

Frigidity

▷ *See* **Sexual Disorders.**

Frostbite

If any part of your body is frostbitten, try the following treatment:
SECALE CORNUTUM 9 C, three pellets three times a day. Apply a few drops of HYPERICUM PERFORATUM M.T. locally.

Functional diseases

Functional diseases are ones in which the symptoms are not due to damage or structural defect of an organ but rather to a problem in the way a normal organ functions or works. A migraine headache, for example, is a disorder which is located in a healthy organ, the brain.
Homeopathy can be particularly effective in treating functional diseases; note that the opposite of functional diseases is organic diseases. (see **Organic diseases**).

Future of Homeopathy (The)

The future of Homeopathy looks bright, thanks to thousands of satisfied patients. Whenever large numbers of people are pleased, they let that be known.
Homeopathy, as a valid discipline of modern medicine, is making positive inroads into public and professional acceptance. Its use as a non-toxic and bona fide therapy, whenever chemical or surgical treatment is unnecessary, is both justified and in the best interests of good health maintenance.

Gait

Unbalanced gait, or the feeling of reeling while standing or walking, may be treated by taking:
ARGENTUM NITRICUM 9 C,
three pellets three times a day.

Gallstones

▷ *See* **Calculi.**

Gas

For gas in the upper digestive tract:
▷ *see* **Eructation.**

For gas in the lower digestive tract:
▷ *see* **Flatulence.**

Gastritis, gastralgia

▷ *See* **Stomach.**

Gastroenteritis

Gastroenteritis is an inflammation of the lining membrane of the stomach or the intestines. It is frequently of infectious origin. Its main symptoms are stomach pains with diarrhea and vomiting.
If the sufferer is an adult or an older child, see the sections: **Stomach** and **Diarrhea.**
If the patient is a baby, check with a doctor.

Gelsemium sempervirens

Base substance: Jessamine or yellow jasmine.

Suitable for:
The shock of bad news; anticipatory anxiety or fear; slowly erupting rashes.

Characteristic signs and symptoms:
Emotional sensitivity; a general slowing down of all activities; worry caused by thinking about a coming event; obnubilation (cloudy thinking); trembling in the extremities; trembling of the tongue; muscular uncoordination; congested face; headache in the occipital region (back of the head) with a feeling that the eyelids are very heavy; diarrhea caused by worrying about a coming event; lack of thirst; fever accompanied by exhaustion and bouts of trembling; rashes or blemishes slow in erupting (accompanied by the above symptoms).

Main clinical uses:
Various types of fever; flu-like symptoms with overall weakness, shivering, stiffness and heaviness of the limbs; coryza; dread; emotional sensitivity; migraine headaches which radiate to the neck and shoulders; the early stages of measles.

WARNING: If condition worsens or persists for more than 72 hours, check with your physician.

German measles

WARNING: Check with a doctor.
Once you're sure of the diagnosis, you may give the child:
PULSATILLA 9 C,
SULPHUR 9 C,
alternate three pellets of each, three times a day for a week.

Germs (Bacteria)

Generally speaking, Homeopathy can provide a treatment for germs, wherever they are in the body. The treatment will not be chosen in accordance with the type of germ involved but rather with the particular symptoms that it causes in the patient.

▷ *See* **Antibiotics.**

Giddiness

▷ *See* **Vertigo.**
A child suffering from fever may feel dizzy. Check with your doctor if symptoms persist.

Gingivitis

▷ *See* **Mouth.**

Glands (Disease of the)

Whenever glandular ailments have a functional origin (see **Functional diseases**), Homeopathy may be very effective. When gland problems are of organic origin (see **Organic diseases**), however, Homeopathy can only reduce the symptoms or slow down the progress of the disease. Ask your homeopathic doctor for advice.

▷ *See* **Addison's disease, Thyroid gland.**

Glaucoma

Glaucoma is damage to the eye caused by abnormally high pressure of the fluid inside the eye. It must be treated by an eye doctor. If you can, find an ophthalmologist specializing in Homeopathy.
Until you can be seen by a doctor, start taking:
> BELLADONNA 5 C,
> SPIGELIA 5 C,
> alternate three pellets of each, three times a day.

Globules

▷ *See* **Pellets, Homeopathic medicines.**

Glonoinum

Base substance: Trinitin or nitroglycerin.

Suitable for:
The consequences of sunstroke; menopause.

Characteristic signs and symptoms:
Headache with sudden rushes of blood to the head, a pounding sensation in the carotid arteries; the person may be confused—for instance, he or she may get lost in familiar streets; symptoms aggravated by the sun and by heat in general.

Main clinical uses:
Congestive migraine; cerebral congestion; menopause; palpitations.

Gluten Intolerance
(Celiac disease)

An illness of young children caused by an intestinal intolerance to gluten (wheat gum, a nitrogenous insoluble cereal protein). Your pediatrician will probably prescribe a gluten-free diet, and fatty diarrhea will disappear with a return to a normal growth curve. The homeopathic physician can

103

prescribe a complementary treatment to speed up the cure. LYCOPODIUM CLAVATUM, PHOSPHORUS and SILICEA are the most commonly prescribed remedies for this disease.

Goiter

▷ See **Thyroid gland.**

Gout

Gout can be treated by Homeopathy. This ailment is caused by collection of crystals of uric acid inside a joint; pain, redness and swelling result. It most frequently occurs in the big toe or in the knee.

For an acute attack:
> BELLADONNA 9 C,
> COLCHICUM AUTUMNALE 9 C,
> NUX VOMICA 9 C,
> alternate three pellets of each, every hour until symptoms have disappeared.

For recurring bouts, see your homeopathic physician.

Granules

▷ See **Pellets, Homeopathic medicines.**

Graphites

Base substance: Plumbago or carbo mineralis.

Suitable for:
Anemic, obese people with unhealthy looking skin. These people have a tendency to shyness and cry easily.

Characteristic signs and symptoms:
Oozing eruptions that look like honey, particularly in flexor folds of the skin

and behind the ears; induration of the skin; badly-healed scars; cracking of the skin (the inside of the cracks look as if they were full of honey); eyelids that stick together in the morning; thick, deformed nails; constipation with large mucus-covered stools; late menstrual periods with flow of light-colored blood.

Main clinical uses:
Weeping eczema; erysipelas; cradle cap; impetigo; badly-healed scars; blepharitis (inflammation of the eyelids).

Grave's disease

▷ See **Thyroid gland.**

Grinding of teeth

▷ See **Teeth.**

Groin

Swollen lymph nodes in the groin:
> MERCURIUS SOLUBILIS 9 C,
> three pellets three times a day.

WARNING: Consult your physician if the swollen nodes do not become smaller after the treatment. If a swollen gland is extremely painful, see your doctor.

Hernia: ▷ see this entry.

Pains in the groin:
> BERBERIS VULGARIS 9 C,
> three pellets three times a day.

Group of Symptoms

This is a concept of utmost importance in Homeopathy.

▷ See **Symptom.**

Growth

Slow growth:
CALCAREA CARBONICA 9 C,
SILICEA 9 C,
alternate three pellets of each,
three times a day, two weeks a
month.

▷ *Also see* **Rickets.**

To keep a child strong who grows too
quickly:
CALCAREA PHOSPHORICA 9 C,
three pellets three times a day, for
one or two months.

Growth epiphysitis

▷ *See* **Scheuermann's disease.**

Gums

▷ *See* **Mouth.**

Gynecology
(Homeopathy in the field of)

Gynecological disorders of functional
origin (see **Functional diseases**) may
be treated by Homeopathy,
particularly disorders related to
menstrual periods. Gynecological
diseases of infectious origin may
sometimes also be treated by
homeopathic medication, but check
with your doctor. **Organic diseases**
(see this entry) can be slowed down by
Homeopathy.
An adult woman should be seen by a
gynecologist at least once a year. Some
gynecologists use Homeopathy.

▷ *Also see* **Menstrual periods,**
Ovaries.

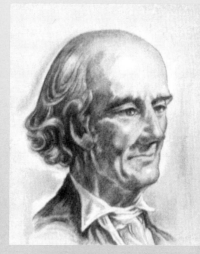

Samuel Hahnemann (1755-1843),
the founder of Homeopathy.

H

"In order to bring about prompt, gentle, and lasting improvement, you most often need to use infinitesimal doses."

SAMUEL HAHNEMANN

Hahnemann
(Christian Samuel)

Samuel Hahnemann (1755-1843) was the true founder of Homeopathy. In 1790 he rediscovered the Law of Similars (see **Homeopathic theory**) and brought it into widespread medical use. His motto was *"Let similars cure similars"* (In Latin, "Similia similibus curentur"). Hahnemann did not take long to discover that infinitesimal potencies (see **Homeopathic theory**) led to even faster and more thorough cures. His fundamental work, *The Organon of the Art of Healing,* was published in Germany in 1810. Hahnemann was born in Saxony and died in Paris, where he is buried.

▷ *See* **History of Homeopathy.**

Hair

Brittle hair:
FLUORICUM ACIDUM 9 C,
three pellets three times a day until improvement.

Hair loss, also known as alopecia (baldness):
PHOSPHORICUM ACIDUM 9 C,
three pellets three times a day.

▷ *See below: Patchy baldness.*

Greasy hair:
PHOSPHORICUM ACIDUM 9 C,
three pellets three times a day.
You should try not to wash your hair more than once a week. The more you wash it, the more sebum or grease is produced and secreted by the glands of the scalp. If you're now washing your hair more than once a week and having problems with greasy hair, getting back to a once weekly wash will make your hair healthier. You can start by progressively leaving a longer time between each shampoo.

Patchy baldness:
FLUORICUM ACIDUM 9 C,
three pellets three times a day.

Dandruff:
Dandruff is only a symptom, not a diagnosis in itself: dandruff may be due to **mycosis, psoriasis** (see these entries), or **seborrhea** (see below). It is therefore a good idea to talk to your doctor about it.
When there is no apparent reason for the dandruff, take:
PHOSPHORICUM ACIDUM 9 C,
three pellets three times a day.

Excess secretion from the scalp glands (seborrhea):
NATRUM MURIATICUM 9 C,
OLEANDER 9 C,
PHOSPHORICUM ACIDUM 9 C,
alternate three pellets of each, three times a day, twenty days a month.

Dry hair:
THUJA OCCIDENTALIS 9 C,
three pellets three times a day.

Hallucinations

Homeopathy cannot treat hallucinations.

Hallux valgus

▷ *See* **Bunions.**

Hamamelis virginica

Base substance: Witch Hazel (also known as spotted or striped Alder).

Characteristic signs and symptoms: Congestion in the veins and painful varicose veins (painful bruising); dark blood when bleeding occurs; inflammation of the testicles.

Main clinical uses:
Varicose veins, orchitis; *WARNING - These diseases are serious. Contact your physician immediately for treatment recommendation.*
Hemorrhoids; various skin ulcerations.

Hands

For rheumatism of the hands, see **Rheumatism.** If you suffer from disfiguring rheumatism, you may supplement your regular treatment with the following:
KALI IODATUM 9 C,
three pellets three times a day.

Hardening of the Arteries

▷ *See* **Arteriosclerosis.**

Hay fever

Take:
ARSENICUM ALBUM 9 C,
HISTAMINUM 9 C,
SABADILLA 9 C,
alternate three pellets of each, three times a day on a regular basis during pollen season.
Depending on symptoms, you may need to add the following:
• if your eyes are irritated,
APIS MELLIFICA 9 C.
• if you sneeze too much,
NUX VOMICA 9 C.
• for accompanying asthma attacks,
IPECAC 9 C.
Apply a small amount of CALENDULA ointment in each nostril every time you go outside.

Headache

Take three pellets of each medicine you select below every half hour. If you need two or three remedies, alternate them every half hour, taking three pellets each time.

Depending on the cause of the headache:
• too much exposure to the heat,
ANTIMONIUM CRUDUM 9 C.
• a cold bath,
ANTIMONIUM CRUDUM 9 C.
• catching cold,
BELLADONNA 9 C.
• a haircut,
BELLADONNA 9 C.
• constipation,
BRYONIA ALBA 9 C.
• intellectual overwork,
CALCAREA PHOSPHORICA 9 C.
• cold and wet weather,
DULCAMARA 9 C.
• sunburn,
GLONOINUM 9 C.
• strong odors,
IGNATIA AMARA 9 C.
• menopause,
LACHESIS 9 C.
• missing a meal,
LYCOPODIUM CLAVATUM 9 C.
• annoyance,
NATRUM MURIATICUM 9 C.
• mild trauma to the head, (See your doctor for head trauma.)
NATRUM SULPHURICUM 9 C.
• overeating,
NUX VOMICA 9 C.
• eyestrain,
ONOSMODIUM 9 C.
• getting wet,
RHUS TOXICODENDRON 9 C.
• muscle fatigue,
RHUS TOXICODENDRON 9 C.

Depending on the circumstances accompanying a headache:
Improved by:
• a cool compress to the head,
ALOE SOCOTRINA 9 C.
• a band around the head,
ARGENTUM NITRICUM 9 C.

- walking,
  PULSATILLA 9 C.
- a warm compress,
  SILICEA 9 C.
- if there happens to be an accompanying nosebleed (you must be seen by a doctor if there is a nosebleed with your headache),
  MELILOTUS OFFICINALIS 9 C.

Made worse by:
- menstrual periods,
  CIMICIFUGA RACEMOSA 9 C.
- noise and light,
  BELLADONNA 9 C.
- coughing,
  BRYONIA ALBA 9 C.
- moving, even such a slight movement as eyeblinking,
  BRYONIA ALBA 9 C.
- motion or riding in a car,
  COCCULUS INDICUS 9 C.
- drinking coffee,
  NUX VOMICA 9 C.
- the weather before a storm,
  PHOSPHORUS 9 C.
- meals (worse after eating),
  PULSATILLA 9 C.
- drafts of air,
  SILICEA 9 C.
- drinking tea,
  THUJA OFFICINALIS 9 C.
- drinking wine,
  ZINCUM METALLICUM 9 C.

Depending on the sensation accompanying a headache:
- a sensation that the head is about to burst (pressure),
  CIMICIFUGA RACEMOSA 9 C.
- throbbing,
  BELLADONNA 9 C.
- a nail driven inside the head,
  COFFEA CRUDA 9 C.
- heavy eyelids,
  GELSEMIUM SEMPERVIRENS 9 C.
- throbbing in the carotid arteries,
  GLONOINUM 9 C.
- hammers beating inside the head,
  NATRUM MURIATICUM 9 C.
- eyes being pulled inwards,
  PARIS QUADRIFOLIA 9 C.

Depending on the localization of the headache pain:
- at the top of the head,
  CIMICIFUGA RACEMOSA 9 C.
- in the temples,
  BELLADONNA 9 C.
- in the entire right half of the head,
  BELLADONNA 9 C.
- in the back of the skull (occiput),
  GELSEMIUM SEMPERVIRENS 9 C.
- alternating pain from one side of the head to the other,
  LAC CANINUM 9 C.
- above the right eye,
  SANGUINARIA CANADENSIS 9 C.
- above the left eye,
  SPIGELIA 9 C.
- the entire left half of the head,
  SPIGELIA 9 C.

Depending on the accompanying symptoms of a headache:
- headache with thirst,
  BRYONIA ALBA 9 C.
- need to urinate,
  GELSEMIUM SEMPERVIRENS 9 C.
- visual disturbances,
  IRIS VERSICOLOR 9 C.
- vomiting that burns,
  IRIS VERSICOLOR 9 C.
- ruddy, congested face and bleeding of the nose,
  MELILOTUS OFFICINALIS 9 C.
- watering or tearing of the eyes,
  PULSATILLA 9 C.
- shivering, shakes or cold sensitivity,
  SILICEA 9 C.
- increased throbbing of the heart,
  SPIGELIA 9 C.
- much diarrhea,
  VERATRUM ALBUM 9 C.
- cold sweats,
  VERATRUM ALBUM 9 C.

▷ *Also see* **Migraines.**

Health (Good)

For the homeopathic physician, good health is a state of balance between external aggressive forces attacking the body and the body's internal defense system. Good health is also the disappearance of symptoms without creating other symptoms (and not merely covering them up with tranquilizers, aspirin or a cream).

Heartburn

▷ *See* **Stomach.**

Heel (Pain in the)

Take:
RHUS TOXICODENDRON 9 C,
three pellets three times a day.

▷ *Also see* **Blisters.**

Helleborus niger

Base substance: Black hellebore or Christmas rose.

Characteristic signs and symptoms:
The person may look dazed, and does not react normally; he or she is apathetic and stares fixedly and frowns; the lower jaw hangs loosely; loss of control of muscles; convulsions; agitated cries during fever; small amounts of urine passed; swollen skin and fetid breath.

Main clinical uses:
Encephalitis, meningitis, and their aftereffects: *WARNING - These diseases are extremely serious. You must contact your physician immediately for treatment recommendation.*

Helonias dioica

Base substance: the Unicorn plant (also known as Starwort).

Characteristic signs and symptoms:
Sudden congestive pain of the uterus; prolapse of the uterus; a hot sensation in or around the kidneys; general fatigue; symptoms relieved by distracting attention.

Main clinical uses:
Prolapse of organs: *WARNING - This disease is serious. Contact your physician immediately for treatment recommendation.*
Fatigue.

Helleborus niger

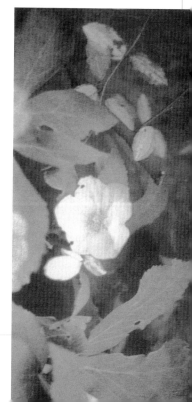

Hematoma

▷ *See* **Injuries.**

Hemophilia

The treatment of hemophilia is not within the realm of Homeopathy. Certain congenital problems of the blood make this impossible. Nevertheless, patients suffering from hemophilia will benefit and have less bruising from the following treatment:
 PHOSPHORUS 9 C,
 three pellets once a day, twenty days per month.

Hemorrhagic proctocolitis

Inflammation of the rectum and intestine, often with much stooling and discharge of blood and mucus.

WARNING: Anytime you see blood in your stools, you must notify your physician.

A homeopathic treatment may be available. In case of a sudden flare-up and in accordance with your physician, take three pellets of:
 MERCURIUS CORROSIVUS 9 C,
 every hour.

Hemorrhoids

To treat hemorrhoids, take:
 AESCULUS HIPPOCASTANUM 3 C,
 HAMAMELIS VIRGINICA 3 C,
 alternate three pellets of each, three times a day for discomfort.

A **local treatment** may be helpful; check with your doctor. Most homeopathic pharmacists offer ointments or suppositories containing AESCULUS, HAMAMELIS, and/or COLLINSONIA CANADENSIS.

For other complications:
- if a fistula forms, take:
 BERBERIS VULGARIS 9 C,
 SILICEA 9 C,
 alternate three pellets of each, three times a day.
- if a hemorrhoid clot forms, take:
 LACHESIS 5 C,
 three pellets three times a day depending on pain. See your doctor if symptoms continue.
- if anal cracking appears, take:
 GRAPHITES 9 C,
 NITRICUM ACIDUM 9 C,
 RATANHIA 9 C,
 alternate three pellets of each, three times a day.

WARNING: If condition persists, discontinue use of the above remedies and consult your physician.

Hepar sulphuris calcareum

Base substance: a Preparation based on flowers of sulfur *(Sulphur)* and the middle layer of the oyster shell *(Calcarea carbonica).*

Suitable for:
Impulsive, easily-irritated individuals who tend to faint.

Characteristic signs and symptoms:
Skin and mucous membrane infections; foul-smelling pus; sharp pains made worse by touch or exposure to cool air; need to consume acidic food; a hoarse cough; sensitivity to cold air.

Main clinical uses:
Minor unresolved suppurative skin conditions, such as eruptions or boils, or the early stages of croupy coughs.

WARNING: If condition worsens or persists for more than 72 hours, check with your physician.

Hepatic

Hepatic insufficiency,
▷ *see* **Liver.**

Hepatic colic,
▷ *see* **Colic.**

Hering (Constantine)

Constantine Hering (1800-1880), a physician of German origin, was one of the first North American homeopaths and is generally considered the father of Homeopathy in America. He was a pupil of Hahnemann's and the founder of the first schools and hospitals in which Homeopathy was taught in the United States. He is particularly well known in connection with the founding of the Hahnemann Medical College and the Homeopathic Medical College of Philadelphia, as well as the American Institute of Homeopathy, which is still an active homeopathic organization today.

He is the author of a great many books, the most famous of which is *Guiding Symptoms,* an extensive Materia Medica consisting of 10 volumes of 500 pages each. He conducted the provings of many homeopathic remedies that are often prescribed in homeopathic practice, such as Lachesis, a South American snake venom.

▷ *See* **History of Homeopathy.**

Hernia

The pain caused by a hiatal hernia (part of the stomach slides up through the diaphragm) may be relieved by:
ARGENTUM NITRICUM 9 C,
three pellets before each meal.

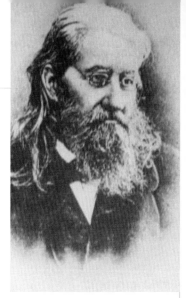

C. Hering
(1800-1880)

This treatment is good for life, each time you have pain.

Surgery for hernia will only be undertaken if the symptoms are severe and particularly painful.

An inguinal hernia must be treated by surgery.

A herniated disk (of a vertebral body in the spine) cannot be treated with Homeopathy. You must be examined by a bone doctor (orthopedist).

Herpes

Herpes, cold sores, or "fever blisters" may occur even without fever. These annoying viral-caused blisters of the mouth and lips often flare up when the body is undergoing a period of stress or weakness (overwork,

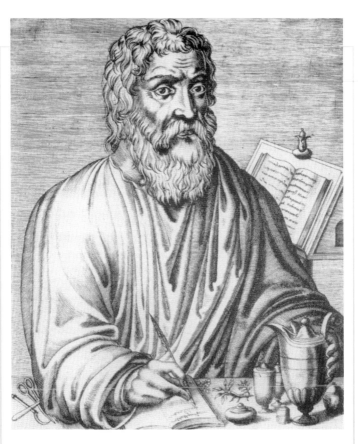

*"By the similars
we prescribe,
the ill do their good health find anew.
Thus whatever suffers little urine
to pass removes that which has already
suffered little urine to pass."*

HIPPOCRATES

emotional upsets, menstrual periods or fever).

For an acute attack, take:
RHUS TOXICODENDRON 9 C,
three pellets three times a day.
Apply locally one or two drops of CALENDULA M.T., three times a day.

A long-term treatment should be worked out between you and your homeopathic physician to prevent or at least reduce the frequency of relapses. NATRUM MURIATICUM and SEPIA are the most commonly-prescribed terrain remedies for herpes.

For circinate herpes,
see **Mycosis.**

Herpes zoster

▷ *See* **Shingles.**

Hiccups

For hiccups, take:
CUPRUM METALLICUM 9 C,
HYOSCYAMUS NIGER 9 C,
alternate three pellets of each, every two minutes until hiccups stop.
If hiccups occur as the result of overeating, you should also use NUX VOMICA 9 C (three pellets crushed or dissolved in mineral water, taken alternately with the above two medicines).
This treatment is suitable for children as well.

Hippocrates

Even Hippocrates wrote about the Law of Similars.

▷ *See* **History of Homeopathy.**

Hips

For pain in the hips, see **Rheumatism.** Once you've selected the appropriate treatment, supplement it with the following:
ALLIUM SATIVUM 9 C,
three pellets three times a day.

History of Homeopathy

Some of the most important names in the history of Homeopathy are:

HIPPOCRATES (460-377 B.C.), more or less the forerunner of Homeopathy because he observed two ways of healing disease: one by using opposites and another by using similars.

PARACELSUS (1493-1541) was well aware of this duality. He treated diarrhea with hellebore, knowing that this substance can also cause diarrhea. He administered very small doses, the equivalent of 1/24th of a drop. Homeopathy now goes much further where diluting of medicines is concerned and is not as esoteric as the work of Paracelsus.

SAMUEL HAHNEMANN (1755-1843) was the true founder of Homeopathy. In 1790 he rediscovered the Law of Similars (see **Homeopathic theory**) and brought it into widespread medical use. His motto was "Let similars cure similars" (In Latin, "Similia similibus curentur"). Hahnemann did not take long to discover that infinitesimal potencies (see **Homeopathic theory**) led to even faster and more thorough cures. His fundamental work, *The Organon of the Art of Healing,* was published in Germany in 1810. Hahnemann was born in Saxony and died in Paris, where he is buried.

CONSTANTINE HERING (1800-1880), a physician of German origin, was one of the first North American homeopaths. He was a pupil of Hahnemann's and the founder of the first schools and hospitals in which Homeopathy was taught in the United States. He is particularly well known in connection with the founding of the Hahnemann Medical College and the Homeopathic Medical College of Philadelphia, as well as the American Institute of Homeopathy, which is still an active homeopathic organization today.

He is the author of a great many books, the most famous of which is *Guiding Symptoms,* an extensive Materia Medica consisting of 10 volumes of 500 pages each. He conducted the provings of many homeopathic remedies that are often prescribed in homeopathic practice, such as Lachesis, a South American snake venom.

C.M. VON BOENNINGHAUSEN (1785-1864), a lawyer who, on becoming cured by Homeopathy, obtained the right to practice Homeopathy in his native province in the Netherlands. He was the author of the first Homeopathic Repertory (see **Repertory**).

JAMES TYLER KENT (1849-1916), an American homeopath, author, and educator. His Repertory is a useful tool to many practitioners throughout the world. His pupils included the great English homeopaths, Margaret Tyler, Douglas Borland, Fergie Woods, and Sir John Weir, the Royal Physician. His American pupils kept Homeopathy alive in the U.S. when it had ceased being taught in medical schools in the mid 1920's.

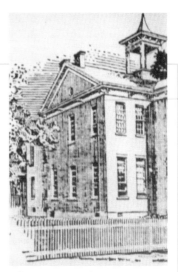

*Allentown, Pennsylvania
(1st homeopathic school in the world)*

History of Homeopathy in the U.S.

Homeopathy was first introduced to the United States in the late 1820's by Dr. Hans Burch Gram. Many of the first homeopaths were German-immigrant or German-American physicians, who had studied directly with Hahnemann, and throughout the century they remained the leaders of the profession. One of the most prominent was Constantine Hering (see above). Supported by successful results in treating cholera and yellow fever epidemics and backed by the press of the time, Homeopathy enjoyed wide public acceptance and won increasing numbers of adherents after the 1850's. It was especially popular for children and city dwellers and was often patronized by clergymen and prominent social figures.

117

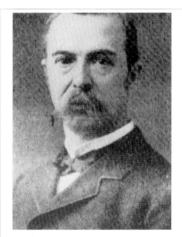

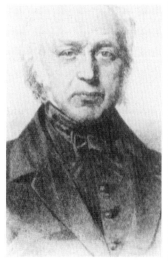

T.F. Allen
(Circa 1880)

C.M. von Boenninghausen
(1785-1864)

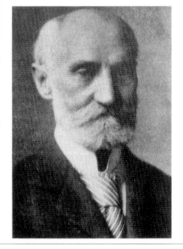

H.C. Allen
(Circa 1890)

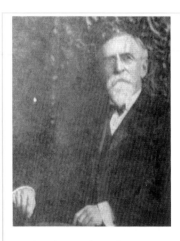

The American Institute of Homeopathy, founded in 1844, was the first national medical association in the United States. By the late 1800's, there were 22 homeopathic medical schools, over 100 homeopathic hospitals, and some 9,500 homeopathic practitioners in the U.S. (of a total of some 50,000 physicians.)

Some of the reasons given for the eventual decline of Homeopathy after the turn of the century are:

1) opposition from the A.M.A. [American Medical Association] and its influence in restricting legislation,
2) failure on the part of the homeopaths to financially support their professional organizations,
3) internal disputes within the second generation of homeopaths, and

E.B. Nash
(Circa 1900)

4) problems with the new influential pharmaceutical companies.

The final blow came in 1910 with the Flexner Report concerning the reform of Schools of Medicine: 17 homeopathic schools were obliged to close. The lean years lasted from 1920 through the 1960's.

By the early 1970's, a timid but evident revival took place. Today homeopathic medical societies are being revived and there is new interest in various areas of homeopathic research. The public's current enthusiasm for Homeopathy lies mainly in the fact that homeopathic remedies are safe, natural and effective and that this individualized therapy encourages a cooperative relationship between doctor and patient.

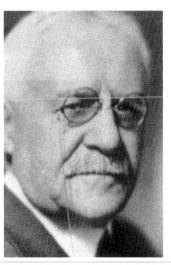

H.A. Roberts
(Circa 1935)

Hoarseness

▷ *See* **Laryngitis.**

Hodgkin's disease

This malignant disease must, and can often now, be effectively treated by specialized, regular physicians (oncologists).

Check with a homeopathic doctor if you are suffering from some of the aftereffects of Hodgkin's disease.

Homeopathic consultation (The)

A general description of a visit to a homeopathic physician.

The doctor will begin by asking a series of questions. Like all doctors, he or she will first try to uncover the symptoms that will help establish the *clinical diagnosis.*

The next step is determining a *therapeutic diagnosis.* This stage, which differentiates Homeopathy from other disciplines of medicine, consists of determining the symptoms due specifically to a certain patient's individual reaction to an illness. Homeopathy does not set out to cure a stomach ulcer, for example, with a conventional, pre-established therapeutic plan: Homeopathy individualizes treatment. The homeopathic physician determines which treatment is best for John Doe and *his* ulcer and which is best for Jane Smith and *her* ulcer. They may both have ulcers but their symptoms and treatment needs may be quite different. The time devoted to making the therapeutic diagnosis is, therefore, very important in Homeopathy.

The homeopathic doctor will also examine you or your children as any physician, but the homeopath may pay more attention to examining your skin, tongue, nails, scalp, etc. to find a proper remedy (soft nails, for instance, will most likely orient the treatment toward THUJA OCCIDENTALIS).

The homeopathic doctor may also order some laboratory tests and X-rays if they are necessary. The last stage of the visit is one in which the physician writes out a prescription (see **Prescriptions)** and discusses it with the patient.

As you can see, a visit to a homeopathic doctor is like a visit to any other doctor, but it's also different in some ways and depends more on your active participation and dialogue with the doctor.

What should the visit be like from the patient's standpoint?

First of all, you can prepare a homeopathic consultation by reading about Homeopathy. Look at the following headings: **Diseases, Homeopathic medicines, Homeopathic theory, Prescriptions.** When you see your doctor, try to pay close attention to the questions he or she asks. Answer *instinctively,* with simple words that seem best to you to describe your symptoms. Don't say what you think the doctor wants to hear. The doctor may seem to ask some questions for which you don't understand the reason (at least not right away). Be patient and try to answer as honestly and openly as possible, avoiding misleading statements. You may, however, talk about any details you feel are important.

If you think your acne was caused by disappointment in love, say so. If your intestines really feel like there was something alive crawling inside, don't be afraid to say it—just that way! Your doctor won't laugh at you. Quite the opposite, the more personalized you can be about your symptom (in your own vocabulary), the more useful your homeopathic doctor can be to you in establishing the best therapeutic diagnosis.

Finally, about *listening:* Your homeopathic doctor is there to give you good advice about your health care, as well as the correct medicine when you need treatment. Listen to what he or she has to say about you and your family's health habits. If you go to your homeopathic physician prepared and receptive, you can come away with a fresh supply of valuable and timely information that can give you a rational basis for hope and action toward better health.

Homeopathic dentists

There are a growing number of dentists who are using Homeopathy in their treatment of patients. Although the remedies they employ are limited in number, their therapeutic results are quite dramatic.

Homeopathic dentists can prepare patients for dental procedures, help relieve toothaches, and treat minor mouth disorders.

For your convenience, many dental conditions are discussed in this book. You can be referred to a homeopathic dentist by your homeopathic pharmacist. There are also a number of books regarding this subject which are available from the principal homeopathic laboratories and organizations.

▷ *See* **Teeth.**

Homeopathic laboratories

When Homeopathy first came to the U.S. the doctors either imported their remedies from Germany or made their own. The first homeopathic pharmacy was established by J.G. Wesselhoeft in New York City in 1835. Dr. Jacob Sheek and Charles Radermacher established a pharmacy shortly thereafter in Philadelphia. Wesselhoeft sold the New York pharmacy to William Radde in 1841. Radde then bought the Radermacher and Sheek Pharmacy in 1858. When Radde died in 1862, both operations were bought by F.E. Boericke, M.D., in Philadelphia. In 1869, Boericke was joined by his brother-in-law, A.J. Tafel, and the firm of Boericke and Tafel was born. The first branch of B&T was opened in California in 1870 and sold to cousin William Boericke in 1882.

Meanwhile, Dr. Luyties opened a pharmacy in St. Louis, Missouri in 1853 and Dr. Frederick Humphreys opened a pharmacy in New York at about the same time.

Shortly after the turn of the century, two young pharmacists who were working for B&T left to form their own organizations.

John A. Borneman, doctor and pharmacist at the Hahnemann Medical College of Pharmacy, founded the Borneman pharmacy in Philadelphia in 1905. The Borneman laboratories eventually moved to Norwood, Pennsylvania. In 1983, they affiliated with Boiron, the largest distributor of quality homeopathic products in the world.

Roger Ehrhart founded Ehrhart and Karl in 1912.

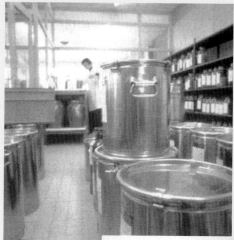

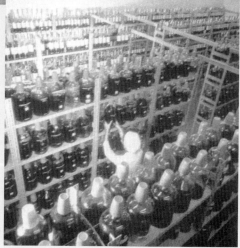

N° 1 The maceration of base substances in alcohol for the preparation of Mother-tinctures. Their storage.

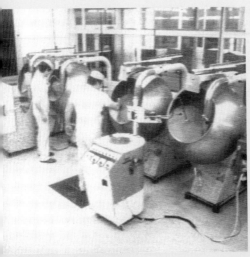

N° 2 The electric turbines used for manufacturing pellets of all sizes.

N° 3 The triple impregnation of pellets by microprocessor is a completely automated operation and insures the high quality level of homeopathic remedies.

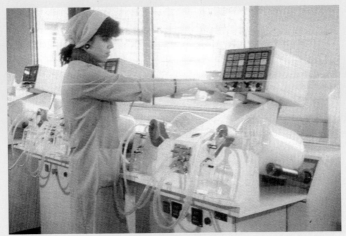

In 1903, Standard Pharmacy in California was founded by a group of doctors and their pharmacist George Hyland. Washington Homeopathic Pharmacy grew out of Mc Pherson's pharmacy, founded in 1873. After serving as the Washington branch of B&T it was sold to C.V. Dorman in 1870. It was bought by W.B. Furr in 1927. In the hands of Furr's son, it moved to Bethesda, Maryland in 1973. Today, all the pharmacies mentioned above are still in business, although a good number of smaller pharmacies and branches of larger ones were forced to shut down during the years following the closing of most of the homeopathic medical schools in this country.[1]

Homeopathic medicines

From where do homeopathic medicines come?

Homeopathic medicines are made from substances derived from one of the three kingdoms of nature. For example:

Vegetable kingdom: NUX VOMICA, the poison nut,

Animal kingdom: CANTHARIS, the Spanish fly,

Mineral kingdom: FERRUM PHOSPHORICUM, ferric phosphate.

How are they made?

Homeopathic medicines are usually made in **laboratories.** The method used is the successive dilution

technique (see **Homeopathic theory, Dilution**). Between each dilution, the product undergoes a series of succussions or vigorous shakings that is known as potentization (see **Potentization**). The medicines are prepared inside a laminar flow air chamber, an extremely clean laboratory hood where the air is virtually particle- and dust-free.

Are homeopathic remedies reliable?

Although the extreme degree of dilution of homeopathic medicines makes their analysis difficult, homeopathic remedies are considered to be extremely reliable due to the strict manufacturing standards of the major homeopathic laboratories.

Are homeopathic medicines toxic?

They are only toxic if not sufficiently diluted. Certain base products, if sold in their undiluted state, would be toxic. (See **Danger in Homeopathy** and the **Appendix: Potency Levels**).

In what forms do homeopathic medicines come?

There are medicated pellets, tablets, mother tinctures (M.T.), drops, etc...

The two typical commercial forms are:
The multi-dose tube:
There are about seventy-five pellets (size 35) in each tube: they are small spherical pills, the size of the heads of a couple of pins. Pellets are generally taken three at a time, by mouth (dissolved under the tongue). The dosage is repeated several times a day according to the doctor's prescription.

The unit-dose tube:
Granules (size 20) are much smaller than pellets: the entire contents of the tube is to be taken all at once. They should be allowed to dissolve under the tongue; for exact dosage, follow your doctor's instructions.

---

1. The author wishes to thank J. Borneman and J. Winston for their kind assistance in providing the above information.

How does the doctor write a homeopathic prescription?

▷ *See* **Prescriptions.**

How should homeopathic remedies be taken?

Pellets, tablets, or drops should be placed directly underneath the tongue and allowed to dissolve. They should not be touched by your fingers. For multi-dose tubes, use the measuring cap on the tube to count the number of pellets you take at one time. (see **When to Take the Medicine You Have Been Prescribed**).

How should homeopathic remedies be stored?

Tubes of pellets and granules may be kept in your medicine chest for several years, but they should not be stored in the same place as camphor (it has a neutralizing, or antidotal effect on the medicine—see **Antidotes and Neutralizers**). A family kit containing the most common homeopathic medicines is easy to select. You should keep a well-stocked one on hand along with *The Guide* (see **Family kit**).

Homeopathic ophthalmologists

Ophthalmologists (eye specialists) may use Homeopathy for treating their patients. Even in this highly specialized field, Homeopathy deserves to play an important role.

▷ *See* **Eyes.**

Homeopathic pediatricians

▷ *See* **Children.**

Homeopathic physician (The)

What is the definition of a homeopathic physician? "A medical doctor who practices Homeopathy exclusively or partially." This means a doctor who has undergone the traditional medical school program and has also been trained in Homeopathy. Homeopathy has become a daily part of his or her medical practice. A homeopathic physician is first of all a doctor, but one who has multiplied his or her abilities to treat patients with the use of Homeopathy.
Very often, a homeopathic physician is a family doctor as well as an advisor, hygienist, counselor, and ecologist.[1]

Homeopathic theory

Homeopathy is based on three main principles: *similarity,* the *infinitesimal,* and a *special concept of the patient and his disease.*

Similarity

The Law of Similars[1] is a universal law of nature. It is the essential basis of Homeopathy and comes out in the etymology of the word "Homeopathy" (see **Etymology**). Its principle is the following: in order to determine which substance will be suitable for a patient, you must first determine, experimentally upon healthy people, which substance causes the same series

---

1. For doctors who wish further information concerning Homeopathy and *homeopathic training programs,* do not hesitate to write to the publisher who will transmit your requests to the author.

of symptoms as those displayed by the patient.

Suppose, for example, that the substance known as Ipecac is being experimented with on healthy people. The symptoms, observed after these healthy subjects have swallowed a small quantity of Ipecac, are: nausea without a coated tongue, a great deal of saliva, coughing accompanied by nausea, a sensation of constrictive discomfort and wheezing in the chest. The sum of these individual symptoms is known as the *experimental symptomatic picture.*

Clinically, a person who has a certain ailment (for example, an asthma sufferer) may display the same group of symptoms, resembling those experimental symptoms described above for Ipecac. This is known as the *clinical symptomatic picture.*

When the experimental and the clinical symptomatic pictures are *similar* (many symptoms in common without being absolutely identical), the Law of Similars can be applied to determine the homeopathic medicine or medicines most appropriate, in this case Ipecac.

The same procedure may be used for prescribing all homeopathic medicines. Each time the patient's symptoms have been correctly observed by the doctor (this is not always easy and depends much on the patient's cooperation), the Law of Similars may be applied.

The Infinitesimal

A full or moderate strength substance prescribed in accordance with the Law of Similars may make the symptoms of an illness worse.

That is why Hahnemann progressively reduced (diluted) the quantity of active drug he was administering. He observed that *"infinitesimal"* doses were quite sufficient to act, and even worked better than stronger doses. (See **History of Homeopathy**).

This concept of "infinitesimal" sometimes boggles the mind. It's difficult to imagine how dilutions containing negligeable amounts of active substance can, in fact, work. That infinitesimal dilutions *are* active is well established by years of clinical observations. And, it follows that *they are active only when the base substance has been correctly chosen according to the Law of Similars.* The infinitesimal, therefore, is a corollary to the Law of Similars.

How are infinitesimal potencies prepared? Starting with the base product which is generally a **mother-tincture** (see this entry), successive dilutions are carried out, using one-hundredth of the previous dilution to start a new one each time. The potencies obtained in this manner are referred to as "Hahnemannian Centesimals" and are abbreviated "C."[2] More specifically, one ml of the base substance mixed with 99 ml of solvent (water + alcohol) gives the "first Hahnemannian Centesimal" or "1 C." To one ml of this 1 C, 99 ml of solvent are added, thus obtaining the "second Hahnemannian Centesimal" or "2 C." This represents a 1/100th dilution of the 1 C, or a 1/10,000th dilution of the base substance. Taking one ml of the 2 C potency and mixing it with 99 ml of more solvent will produce the "3 C" (a one-millionth dilution of the base substance) and so on. (See diagram).

By referring to a theoretical calculation known as **Avogadro's number,** it has been determined that between the 11th and 12th centesimals there is no longer a single molecule of the base substance left in the preparation. The dilution process for the base product has,

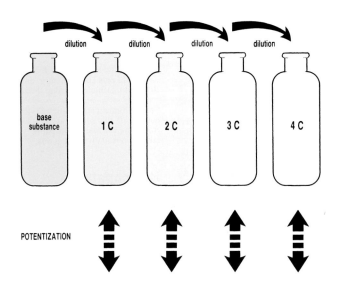

The preparation of homeopathic
centesimal potencies

1 ml of the base substance or mother-tincture is added to 99 ml of vehicle.
After shaking, a 1/100th or 1C potency is obtained.
Subsequent dilutions are made by serial progression, using 1 part of the preceding potency and 99 parts of vehicle.

1 C contains 1 part base substance plus 99 parts of vehicle.

2 C contains 1 part of the 1 C plus 99 parts of vehicle.

3 C contains 1 part of the 2 C plus 99 parts of vehicle,
and so on.

N.B.: This series of dilutions may be carried out according to the same method but to the 10th (1 part base substance or preceding potency for 9 parts vehicle); the potencies are then decimal and are labeled 1 X, 2 X, 3 X, etc.

therefore, been carried out successively beyond Avogadro's number (6.023 X 10^{23}). Once having reached the 12th dilution to the 1/100th, there should be nothing left of the original product, and yet the process is continued even further.

Homeopathy works even if this theoretical limit is crossed. The facts must be accepted even if we don't exactly understand how the mechanism of action works. Doctors' observations of thousands of successfully treated cases is surely more reliable than theory, or rather, ahead of theory. Someday science will be able to explain exactly how Homeopathy works and will expand our knowledge of the infinitesimal (see **Research - Scientific in Homeopathy**). Diluting a medicine is not the only important thing. Potentization, or vigorous shaking of each dilution, is also carried out at each step. Without potentization, the end-product or potency would have no therapeutic activity.

To find out how the homeopathic physician chooses the dilution strength of each remedy, see **Dosage.**

The Homeopathic Perception of the Patient and his Disease—a Special Concept.

Homeopathic remedies are not taken blindly "against" a certain disease.[3] There are no standard recipes, no

single treatment for asthma, eczema, migraine, measles, or any other disease. Homeopathic treatment is individualized, and aims at evoking each person's reactional mode. (See **Reactional Mode**).

Homeopathic veterinarians

Veterinarians may treat both small household pets and large farm animals the homeopathic way, using the same remedies as for humans.

Several homeopathic veterinary books concerning this subject are available from the principal homeopathic laboratories and organizations.

Homeopathy

Etymology:
The word **"Homeopathy"** comes from two Greek words: *homoeo* (similar) and *pathos* (disease). This clearly points to the Law of Similars.

Definition:
Homeopathy is a therapeutic method. It clinically applies the Law of Similars and uses medically active substances at weak or infinitesimal doses.

How Homeopathy works

The precise mechanism of action of Homeopathy is not known. It can be stated, however, that homeopathic remedies stimulate the body's natural defense systems. It is not the quantity of homeopathic medicine that counts, but rather its presence that determines

---

1. There is a difference between "similarity" and "analogy": see **Analogy.**
2. "Hahnemannian decimal potencies" (X) are diluted to the tenth rather than to the hundredth. See **Dilution.**
3. The reader will often have to make a choice about which homeopathic medicines to take, and in such a way adapts Homeopathy to his or her individual needs. There are no ready-made or pat answers.

its activity. **Immunology** (see this entry) will one day help us to discover exactly how homeopathic remedies act.

▷ *Also see* **Dynamism, Homeopathic theory, Reactional Mode.**

Humidity (Sensitivity to)

Take:
THUJA OCCIDENTALIS 9 C,
DULCAMARA 9 C,
alternate three pellets of each, three times a day, for two weeks a month over a period of several months.

Hunger

Lack of hunger, ▷ *see* **Appetite.**

Constant hunger, ravenous hunger, ▷ *see* **Bulimia.**

Hydrarthrosis

▷ *See* **Synovitis.**

Hydrastis canadensis

Base substance: Golden seal.

Characteristic signs and symptoms: Chronic yellow, thick secretions from the mucous membranes; chronic constipation without urge to defecate; sensation of emptiness in the pit of the stomach with dyspepsia, made worse by eating bread; enlarged liver.

Main clinical indications: Hepatic insufficiency; constipation; pharyngitis; *WARNING - These diseases are serious. You should consult your physician for advice.* Sinusitis; dyspepsia; gastritis.

Hygiene and Health Recommendations

The homeopathic physician will be able to *personalize* hygiene, health and nutrition recommendations, basing them on the remedies that are appropriate for you and your family. For example, with NATRUM MURIATICUM, the doctor may advise you to avoid the seaside during warm weather. Since fifty percent of people with symptoms characteristic of NATRUM MURIATICUM become fatigued after one week spent in such climates.

Hygroma

This is a collection of fluid causing swelling, often around a joint (bursitis, housemaid's knee).
Rub with tincture of iodine once or twice (not more, and be careful not to bandage too tightly) then take:
APIS MELLIFICA 9 C,
three pellets, three times a day until symptoms disappear.

Hyoscyamus niger

Base substance: Black henbane.

Characteristic signs and symptoms: Violent delirium with incessant talkativeness and fear of being poisoned; the person takes his or her covers or clothes off, mumbles, grimaces and laughs; muscle spasms; hiccups following meals; coughing as soon as lying down; involuntary passing of stools; enuresis (bedwetting).

Main clinical uses: Delirium caused by fever; convulsions; typhoid fever: *WARNING - These*

diseases are extremely serious. You must contact your physician immediately for treatment recommendation.
Hiccups; coughing.

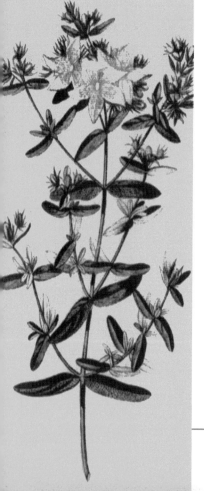

Hypericum perforatum

Base substance: Saint John's wort.

Suitable for:
Trauma of the nerves; wounds around an area of many nerve endings.

Characteristic signs and symptoms:
Pain ascending the length of a nerve, ("ant crawling sensation"), starting from a lacerated wound made worse by touching; pain in the coccyx after falling (pain moves up the spinal column); pain in bunions.

Main clinical uses:
Pain involving the nerve endings; wound pain; pain in the coccyx.

Hyperventilation

Hyperventilation is increased breathing beyond that needed by the body. The blowing off of carbon dioxide leads to a number of symptoms, including tetany or muscle spasms in severe cases.
If someone who is hyperventilating suffers from an attack of tetany (or numbness or "pins and needles" in the extremities), call a doctor and take:
COCCULUS INDICUS 9 C,
three pellets every five minutes or quarter of an hour depending on intensity.
In case of recurring attacks, check with a homeopathic physician (the remedies which are most often prescribed as a terrain treatment are NATRUM MURIATICUM and SEPIA).

Hysteria

▷ *See* **Neurosis.**

Hypericum perforatum

IJK
L

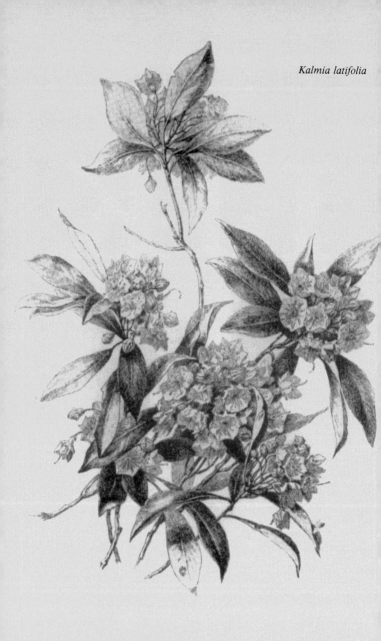

Kalmia latifolia

Iberis amara

Base substance: The seeds of the Bitter candytuft.

Characteristic signs and symptoms:
Palpitations from the slightest movement; irregular pulse; physical awareness of the heart; suffocation; enlarged heart.

Main clinical uses:
Palpitations; extrasystoles; enlarged heart due to nervous causes.

WARNING: As with any heart condition, these diseases are serious. You must consult your physician for treatment recommendation.

Ignatia amara

Base substance: Saint Ignatius bean.

Suitable for:
The effects of emotion, vexation, bereavement or other sad events.

Characteristic signs and symptoms:
A lump in the throat; nervous yawning; decreased respiration with a need to sigh; moodiness; keeping emotions bottled up inside and mulling them over; irritability, contradicting everyone and everything; increased sensitivity to smells, particularly coffee and tobacco; severe pounding migraines; emptiness in the pit of the stomach; sharp erratic pains.

Main clinical indications:
Migraine of nervous origin; minor mental and emotional disorders; muscle spasms from various outside disturbances; rheumatism of nervous origin; contradictory symptoms, i.e., nausea relieved by eating.

WARNING: If condition worsens or persists for more than 72 hours, check with your physician.

Immunology

Immunology, the science of how the body defends itself from disease and infection, is a rapidly developing branch of modern medicine.
The scientific connection between Homeopathy and classical medicine lies in immunology: the body's own natural systems of immunity and how they can be safely called into action.

▷ *See* **Homeopathic theory** and **Terrain.**

Impaction of the bowel

Blockage of the large intestine from impacted stool. This is constipation in the extreme, often accompanied by vomiting, gassiness and abdominal pain. You must see a doctor as soon as possible.
Don't think that you are suffering from impaction of the bowel each time you are simply constipated. Impaction is much rarer.

Impatience

If you're often impatient and anxious (wanting to get everything over with before starting), take:
ARGENTUM NITRICUM 9 C,
three pellets three times a day.
If you're so irritated that you would rather rip off a button than get it right in the buttonhole or if you think that everyone around you should know what you mean as soon as you start to speak, take:
NUX VOMICA 9 C,
three pellets three times a day.

Hurried people who always try to get a job over with before it's even started will benefit from:

ARGENTUM NITRICUM 9 C,
three pellets three times a day over ten-day periods.

▷ *Also see* **Legs** (Restlessness in the).

Impetigo

Impetigo (fluid-filled or crusted skin rashes, of infectious origin, particularly in children) should react favorably to:

GRAPHITES 9 C,
MEZEREUM 9 C,
alternate three pellets of each three times a day.

Topically: apply CALENDULA ointment, once or twice a day.

Impotence

▷ *See* **Sexual disorders.**

Incontinence

Of urine, ▷ *see* **Enuresis.**

Of stools, take:

ALOE SOCOTRINA 9 C,
three pellets three times a day.

Indigestion

▷ *See* **Digestion.**

Individualization

Homeopathy is a field of medicine in which diagnosing and treating people on an individual basis is of primary importance (the Law of Similars requires this principle). Two people with the same disease may not necessarily need the same treatment; this depends on each person's individual symptoms. That's why this book seldom suggests just one medicine for any particular illness or symptom. Based on specific symptoms, the reader can choose what's best for him or her and should always consult a homeopathic doctor when in doubt. Self-treatment with homeopathic medicines requires an attentive and observing attitude toward our own bodies.

Infectious mononucleosis

This is a self-limiting disease (runs its course and disappears) characterized by fever, sore throat, swollen lymph nodes in the neck, and fatigue. It usually occurs in children or young people. See your doctor. A blood test will confirm the diagnosis (presence of too many "mononuclear" white blood cells).

To help diminish tiredness, you may take:

MERCURIUS SOLUBILIS 9 C,
NATRUM MURIATICUM 9 C,
alternate three pellets of each, three times a day. You should take these until fatigue has completely disappeared and your blood tests return to normal.

Infinitesimal

▷ *See* **Homeopathic medicines, Homeopathic theory.**

Influenza
(Flu and flu-like symptoms)

To prevent an attack of influenza, take:
INFLUENZINUM 30 C,
three pellets a week - from October
to April.
The above treatment isn't a vaccine
but it works in a similar way. The
classical vaccine is usually reserved for
the elderly or other patients at risk of
bad flu infections. The following flu
treatments can be used by people who
have not been vaccinated.

Treatment for acute attacks:
SULPHUR 30 C,
one unit-dose tube.
Alternate three pellets of each of the
following remedies three times a day
until the flu symptoms have entirely
disappeared:
EUPATORIUM PERFOLIATUM 9 C,
GELSEMIUM SEMPERVIRENS 9 C,
RHUS TOXICODENDRON 9 C.
Don't confuse flu (an epidemic viral
respiratory illness with high fever,
chills, prostration, muscle aches, dry
cough and headache) with colds
(runny nose and mild fever).

▷ See **Colds.**

Injuries (Minor trauma)

Do not hesitate to see a doctor for
trauma.

General treatment suggestions for minor injuries

Take three pellets of one or more of
the following medicines three times a
day:

Minor burns:
- with pinkish swelling or wheals,
APIS MELLIFICA 9 C.
- with red swelling,
BELLADONNA 9 C.
- with a small blister,
RHUS TOXICODENDRON 9 C.

- with a large blister,
CANTHARIS 9 C.

Scars: ▷ *see* this entry.

Contusions without cuts:
ARNICA MONTANA 9 C.

Cuts: (Stitches may be needed; ask
your doctor.)
- if the edges are clean-cut,
STAPHYSAGRIA 9 C.
- if the edges are ragged and lacerated,
ARNICA MONTANA 9 C.

Sprains:
ARNICA MONTANA 9 C,
RHUS TOXICODENDRON 9 C,
RUTA GRAVEOLENS 9 C,
alternate three pellets of each,
three times a day.

*Mild frostbite, exposure to freezing
temperatures:* (Requires a doctor's
exam.)
SECALE CORNUTUM 9 C.

Hematoma, bruises:
ARNICA MONTANA 9 C.

Minor bleeding from an injury:
ARNICA MONTANA 9 C.
(Check with your doctor if the
bleeding won't stop.)

Insect bites:
APIS MELLIFICA 9 C,
LEDUM PALUSTRE 9 C,
alternate three pellets of each,
three times a day.

*Pricks caused by thorns, needles or
nails:* (Make sure your tetanus
immunization is up-to-date.)
LEDUM PALUSTRE 9 C.

Open wounds:
LEDUM PALUSTRE 9 C.

Local treatment suggestions

As soon as possible after the injury,
apply local compresses of the
following:
- for a blow that doesn't cause an
open wound,
ARNICA MONTANA M.T.
- for an injury resulting in an open
wound or burn,
CALENDULA M.T.

135

• for frostbite or exposure to freezing temperatures,
> HYPERICUM PERFORATUM M.T.
• for pricks or insect bites,
> LEDUM PALUSTRE M.T.
• for sprains,
> RHUS TOXICODENDRON M.T.
> (use just once, the first day).

▷ *Also see* **Trauma (Minor).**

Insanity

Insanity cannot be treated by Homeopathy. See a doctor.

Insect bites

For insect bites or stings, take:
> APIS MELLIFICA 9 C,
> LEDUM PALUSTRE 9 C,
> alternate three pellets of each, every half hour or hour.

People who are allergic to insect bites or stings would do well to always carry these two products with them and in case of a bite or sting, alternate them every two minutes while seeking medical help.
> LEDUM PALUSTRE M.T.,
> should be applied locally. (Use two or three drops a day).
> LEDUM PALUSTRE 9 C,
> can also help prevent bee stings.

Beekeepers who take three pellets a few minutes before working around their hives will notice a marked drop in the number of stings.

Insomnia

Newly occurring insomnia reacts very positively to Homeopathy. Depending on the circumstances, take three pellets of one of the following remedies at bedtime (repeat this dose

after a half an hour if necessary or if you should wake up in the middle of the night).
• insomnia caused by being frightened,
> ACONITUM NAPELLUS 9 C.
• during menstrual periods,
> CIMICIFUGA RACEMOSA 9 C.
• due to worry,
> ARSENICUM ALBUM 9 C.
• insomnia despite the desire to go to sleep,
> BELLADONNA 9 C.
• unpleasant images when closing your eyes,
> BELLADONNA 9 C.
• insomnia caused by loss of vital body fluids (from diarrhea, vomiting, heavy perspiration),
> CINCHONA OFFICINALIS 9 C.
• due to the presence of worms in the intestines,
> CINA 9 C.
• from staying up too late,
> COCCULUS INDICUS 9 C.
• from too much thinking,
> COFFEA CRUDA 9 C.
• from drinking too much coffee,
> COFFEA CRUDA 9 C.
• after hearing some good news,
> COFFEA CRUDA 9 C.
• because of neuralgia (or pain in a nerve somewhere),
> COFFEA CRUDA 9 C.
• because you are afraid you can't sleep,
> GELSEMIUM SEMPERVIRENS 9 C.
• after hearing some bad news,
> GELSEMIUM SEMPERVIRENS 9 C.
• after an upsetting emotional disturbance,
> IGNATIA AMARA 9 C.
• from intellectual strain,
> KALI PHOSPHORICUM 9 C.
• because of muscle cramps,
> NUX VOMICA 9 C.
• after drinking too much alcohol,
> NUX VOMICA 9 C.
• after eating too much,
> NUX VOMICA 9 C.
• from physical stress or muscular fatigue,
> RHUS TOXICODENDRON 9 C.

- for a child who is afraid of the dark and has to keep a light on,
  STRAMONIUM 9 C.
- because the child's feet are hot and must be uncovered to cool them off,
  SULPHUR 9 C.
- because the child can't sleep if there is the slightest noise, even the dropping of a pin,
  THERIDION 9 C.
- because of a constant need to move the legs,
  ZINCUM METALLICUM 9 C.

Insomnia in longtime sufferers is difficult to treat except in people who have tremendous willpower. Here is how to try: do away with all chemical sleeping pills. Don't take any other sleeping medicine except the homeopathic medicines listed above. For several nights you may not sleep at all; but, one night, natural sleep will come again. This treatment may be difficult to follow and does not suit everyone. Those who try it, however, may find they can get rid of the bad habit of taking pills to sleep. It might be best to try this treatment when you're on vacation.
The best treatment, of course, is not to start taking sleeping pills! It becomes a habit that's hard to break. It's better not to sleep a night or two than to become dependent on sleeping medication.

Intercostal pain
(Pain between the ribs)

For intercostal pain, take:
  BRYONIA ALBA 9 C,
  RANUNCULUS BULBOSUS 9 C,
  alternate three pellets of each,
  three times a day until pain stops.
If pain continues, or if you think you might have injured a rib, see your doctor.

Intertrigo

Infection of the folds of the skin. This is often due to a mild yeast infection of a humid area (underarms, groin, between toes, etc.).

Intertrigo may be treated with the following remedies:
  GRAPHITES 9 C,
  HEPAR SULPHURIS CALCAREUM 9 C,
  alternate three pellets of each,
  three times a day.

Locally: Apply CALENDULA M.T. to affected areas twice a day.

Intestines

▷ *See* **Constipation, Diarrhea, Flatulence, Gastroenteritis.**

Intoxication by Alcohol

In case of an occasional intoxication by alcohol:
  AGARICUS MUSCARIUS 9 C,
  NUX VOMICA 9 C,
  alternate three pellets of each,
  every five minutes.

Iodium

Base substance: Iodine.

Suitable for:
Thin, restless individuals with yellowish skin.

Characteristic signs and symptoms:
Constant worry and restlessness; anxiety made worse by resting and by abstaining from eating; the person loses weight despite a good appetite; intolerance to heat; enlarged thyroid gland; light or grayish diarrhea; swollen lymph nodes; irritating mucous secretions.

Main clinical uses:
Goiter; Grave's disease of the thyroid gland; pancreatitis: *WARNING - These diseases are extremely serious. Contact your physician immediately for treatment recommendation.*

Ipecacuanha (or Ipecac)

Base substance: Ipecac root.

Characteristic signs and symptoms:
Constant nausea (tongue remains uncoated); coughing accompanied by nausea; a feeling of constriction inside the chest; shortness of breath; bleeding of bright red blood, particularly from the nose; diarrhea; aggravation of these symptoms by hot, humid wind; annual occurrence of symptoms.

Main clinical uses:
Hay fever; coughing; bronchitis; nausea; indigestion; vomiting; diarrhea; hypersalivation with a clear, non-coated tongue.

WARNING: If condition worsens or persists for more than 72 hours, check with your physician.

Iris versicolor

Base substance: Blue Flag lily.

Characteristic signs and symptoms:
Hyperacidity of the digestive tract with a burning sensation in the mouth, throat, esophagus, stomach, intestines and anus; migraine headaches centered around the eyes and accompanied by burning vomiting.

Main clinical uses:
Migraines around the eyes; migraines with bilious vomiting; pancreatitis.

Iritis

Inflammation of the iris.

▷ *See* **Eyes.**

Irritability

There exist a number of remedies for irritability. Take three pellets of one of the following medicines three times a day (these are the most common ones):

- for irritable children,
    CHAMOMILLA 9 C.
- for irritability with a tendency to be contradictory,
    IGNATIA AMARA 9 C.
- for irritability and impatience,
    NUX VOMICA 9 C.

Isotherapics

Isotherapics, also known as isopathics, allersodes or isodes, are dilutions prepared according to the homeopathic method (see **Homeopathic medicines**) from the very substances which caused the illness in the first place.
This method is rarely used in the United States; consult your physician.

Itching, pruritus

If the itching is due to a particular skin problem, look under the corresponding entry: **Eczema, Psoriasis, Urticaria,** etc.
If the itching is localized and not related to a rash, blister or other lesion of the skin, take one of the following remedies, three pellets three times a day until symptoms disappear.
Itching is classified under four headings:

Origin:
- Itching without apparent cause,
  DOLICHOS PRURIENS 9 C.
- Itching in elderly people,
  DOLICHOS PRURIENS 9 C.
- Itching due to annoyance or aggravation,
  IGNATIA AMARA 9 C.

Modifying circumstances:
Aggravated by:
- alcohol ingestion,
  CHLORALUM HYDRATE 9 C.
- heat,
  DOLICHOS PRURIENS 9 C.
- the night,
  DOLICHOS PRURIENS 9 C.
- contact with wool,
  HEPAR SULPHURIS CALCAREUM 9 C.
- scratching,
  MEZEREUM 9 C.
- the slightest touch,
  RANUNCULUS BULBOSUS 9 C.
- getting undressed,
  RUMEX CRISPUS 9 C.
- the open air,
  RUMEX CRISPUS 9 C.

Ameliorated by:
- heat,
  ARSENICUM ALBUM 9 C.
- bleeding,
  DOLICHOS PRURIENS 9 C.
- cold water,
  FAGOPYRUM ESCULENTUM 9 C.
- scratching,
  RHUS TOXICODENDRON 9 C.

Sensation:
- a burning sensation of the skin relieved by warm compresses,
  ARSENICUM ALBUM 9 C.
- a burning sensation improved by cool compresses,
  SULPHUR 9 C.
- of severe itching,
  MEZEREUM 9 C.
- migrating itching (as soon as you scratch one place, itching starts up in another),
  STAPHYSAGRIA 9 C.
- itching that feels like pin pricks,
  URTICA URENS 9 C.

Accompanying symptoms:
- Itching with disorders of the liver or constipation,
  DOLICHOS PRURIENS 9 C.
- Itching with shivering (can't stand cold weather),
  MEZEREUM 9 C.

A **local treatment** may be necessary; check with your physician.

▷ *Also see* **Anus.**

Jaundice

Yellowing of the skin, or jaundice. Jaundice can have several causes: **viral hepatitis** (see this entry), **gallstones** (see **Calculi**), lesions of the pancreas, etc. You have to check with a doctor if you develop jaundice, no matter what the cause.
There exist several homeopathic remedies that may be right for you.

Jellyfish (Sting of)

If you're stung by a jellyfish, take the following remedies as soon as possible:
  APIS MELLIFICA 9 C,
  MEDUSA 9 C,
  alternate three pellets of each, every five minutes.
If MEDUSA 9 C is not available, replace by:
  URTICA URENS 9 C.
Place a slice of raw tomato on the wound for local relief of stinging.

Joint Pains

▷ *See* **Rheumatism.**

Kali bichromicum

Base substance: Potassium bichromate.

Suitable for:
Inflammation, exudation or ulceration of the mucous membranes.

Characteristic signs and symptoms:
Abundant stringy, sticky, greenish-yellow mucous secretion; crusting inside the nose; loss of sense of smell; speaking voice with nasal quality; polyps in the nose; erratic pains; various types of skin or mucous membrane ulcerations; alternation of rheumatism and diarrhea; burning pain in the stomach, made worse by drinking beer; migraine headaches centered around the eyes.

Main clinical uses:
Rheumatism; sciatica; stomach ulcers; ophthalmic migraine: _WARNING - These diseases are serious. You should consult your physician for advice._ Chronic colds; sinusitis; bronchitis.

Kali bromatum

Base substance: Potassium bromide.

Characteristic signs and symptoms:
General numbness of the nervous system; decrease of intellectual abilities; sadness with an uncontrollable desire to cry; decrease of sexual desire; restlessness, especially of the hands; nightmares; various types of spasms; acne.

Main clinical uses:
Depression; spasms; restlessness; nightmares; enuresis; acne.

Kali carbonicum

Base substance: Potassium carbonate.

Suitable for:
The period following pregnancy (post-partum period); elderly people.

Characteristic signs and symptoms:
Anxiety and pain felt in the stomach; intellectual and physical fatigue; pain in the lumbar region; a tendency to perspire; pricking pains that don't change on movement; irritation of the mucous membranes; bloating of the stomach and abdomen; inflammation of the medial corner of the upper eyelid (nearest the nose).

Main clinical uses:
Asthma; whooping cough: _WARNING - These diseases are serious. You must check with your doctor for treatment recommendation._
Lumbar pain; gout; rheumatism; fatigue; depression.

Kali phosphoricum

Base substance: Potassium phosphate.

Suitable for:
Intellectual strain or overwork.

Characteristic signs and symptoms:
Mental exhaustion; inability to concentrate, accompanied by irritability; nightmares; headaches resulting from intellectual strain; foul-smelling diarrhea; a yellowish tongue.

Main clinical uses:
Minor depression; mental exhaustion; enuresis.

Kalmia latifolia

Base substance: Mountain laurel.

Characteristic signs and symptoms:
Erratic, searing pains shooting down a nerve; sensation of numbness; palpitations; slow pulse.

Main clinical uses:
Neuralgia, especially in the face;
erratic rheumatism.

Kent (James Tyler)

James Tyler Kent (1849-1916), an
American homeopath, author, and
educator. His Repertory is a useful
tool to many practitioners throughout
the world. His pupils included the
great English homeopaths, Margaret
Tyler, Douglas Borland, Fergie Woods,
and Sir John Weir, the Royal
Physician. His American pupils kept
Homeopathy alive in the U.S. when it
ceased being taught in medical schools
in the mid 1920's.

▷ *See* **History of Homeopathy.**

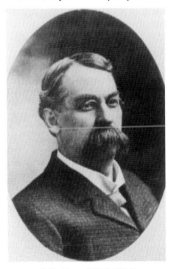

J.T. Kent (1849-1916)

Knees

▷ *Look under* the sections
corresponding to your symptoms
(**Sprains, Rheumatism,** etc.).
You should also add the following to
the treatment you decide upon:
    BENZOICUM ACIDUM 9 C,
      three pellets three times a day.

Korsakov's dilution method

A special way of preparing
homeopathic medicine for low
dilutions. Normally, the diluting
process is carried out in accordance
with the Hahnemannian separate flask
technique (a separate flask for each
new potency). With Korsakov's
method, however, the same flask is
emptied and used over again for the
next dilution: it is felt that a sufficient
amount of the active product
(approximately 1 percent) remains on
the walls of the flask.

▷ *See* **Dilution.**

Kyphosis (Humpback)

Convex curving of the spinal column.

▷ *See* **Spinal Column** for pains caused
by kyphosis.

Lac caninum

Base substance: the Milk of female
dogs.

Characteristic signs and symptoms:
Symptoms that constantly go from one
side of the body to the other
(migraines, throat pains, rheumatism,
pain in the ovaries); swollen breasts,

particularly before menstrual periods; diphtheritic membranes in the throat.

Main clinical uses:
Diphtheria: _WARNING_ - This disease is serious. Contact your physician immediately for treatment recommendation.
Congestion of the breasts; menstrual disorders; rheumatism.

Lachesis

Base substance: the Venom of the American pit viper. (first used by Constantine Hering)

Suitable for: Women undergoing menopause.

Characteristic signs and symptoms:
Nervousness or anxiety in the evening; depression in the morning; dreams about death; talkativeness; extreme sensitivity to touch; sore throat beginning on the left and crossing over to the right, with intolerance to hot liquids and being touched on the neck; hot flashes with violaceous congestion of the skin; a general tendency to bleeding of dark blood; spontaneous (non-traumatic) bruising; general improvement when menstrual period begins; left-sided predominance of all symptoms, or crossing over of symptoms from left to right.

Main clinical uses:
Sore throat; leg ulcers; abscesses; depression; asthma; migraines; various types of bleeding; menopause.

WARNING: If condition worsens or persists for more than 72 hours, check with your physician.

Lachnanthes tinctoria

Base substance: Red Root
Characteristic signs and symptoms:
Pain and stiffness of the neck (torticollis); head leaning to one side.
Main clinical uses:
Rheumatic torticollis (wryneck); sore throat with torticollis: _WARNING - These diseases are serious. Contact your physician immediately for treatment recommendation._

Lapis albus

Base substance: Silico-fluoride of calcium, also known as Gastein Rock.
Main clinical use:
Benign glandular tumors: _WARNING - This disease is serious. Contact your physician immediately for treatment recommendation._

Laryngitis

Acute laryngitis:
Take three pellets of one or two of the following remedies three times a day depending on symptoms (pain and loss of voice are the most frequent).

WARNING: Check with a doctor if the condition has not improved within a few days.

- laryngitis after exposure to dry cold,
  ACONITUM NAPELLUS 9 C.
- laryngitis with the feeling of having a thorn in the throat when swallowing,
  ARGENTUM METALLICUM 9 C.
- laryngitis with partial or total loss of voice after straining the vocal cords,
  ARUM TRIPHYLLUM 9 C.
- sharp pains with voice loss,
  CAUSTICUM 9 C.
- voice loss of anxious or nervous origin,
  IGNATIA AMARA 9 C.

- pain which is worse in the evening, accompanied by hoarseness,
  PHOSPHORUS 9 C.
- voice loss relieved by speaking,
  RHUS TOXICODENDRON 9 C.

Chronic laryngitis: see a doctor.

Laxatives

▷ *See* **Constipation.**

Ledum palustre

Base substance: Wild Rosemary.

Characteristic signs and symptoms:
Swelling of the joints that are cold to the touch; joint pains relieved by bathing in cold water; rheumatism that progresses upward; wounds caused by sharp objects or insects; bruises, particularly around the eyes; black eyes.

Main clinical uses:
Gout: *WARNING - This disease is serious. You should consult your physician for advice.*
Various types of insect bites; acne rosacea; mild injury to the eyes (black eye).

Left-handedness

A definite preference to use the left hand rather than the right should not be something to get upset about, even in children. An adult who worries or feels antagonistic because he was obliged to use his right hand since childhood may be helped by the following:
ARGENTUM NITRICUM 9 C,
three pellets three times a day over a period of ten days (at will).

Legs

A feeling of heaviness in the legs:
HAMAMELIS VIRGINICA 3 C,
AESCULUS HIPPOCASTANUM 3 C,
alternate three pellets of each, three times a day.

Restlessness of the legs; constant need to move the legs; impatient movements of the legs:
ZINCUM METALLICUM 9 C,
three pellets, each time the problem occurs.

▷ *Also see* **Ulcers.**

Lesions

▷ *See* **Organic diseases.**

Leukorrhea

▷ *See* **Vaginal discharge.**

Lice

Body lice is a parasitic infestation that requires special cleansing and eradication. See your doctor. Supplement the usual local treatment with:
PEDICULUS CAPITIS 5 C,
three pellets three times a day.

Lichen

A bumpy skin rash of unknown origin, usually itchy and distributed over flexor surfaces (inside of elbows, back of knees) or in the mouth. See a skin doctor if the condition persists.
Take:
ANACARDIUM ORIENTALE 9 C,
RHUS TOXICODENDRON 9 C,
alternate three pellets of each, three times a day.

If the rash appeared after an emotional shock, supplement the above remedies with:
IGNATIA AMARA 9 C,
three pellets three times a day.

Lilium tigrinum

Base substance: the Tiger lily.

Characteristic signs and symptoms: Emotional breakdown with fits of crying worsened by attempts at consolation; irritability; a constant need to be doing something; sexual excitation; a sensation of heaviness in the lower abdomen; palpitations with a sensation that the heart is in a vise.

Main clinical uses: Nervous or emotional breakdown; uterine cramps; false angina pectoris; sexual overexcitement.

Limits of Homeopathy (The)

Like any other branch of medicine, Homeopathy has its limits. People suffering, for example, from psychosis or organic diseases may no longer be able to react to homeopathic treatment (see **Reactional Mode**).

▷ *Also see* **Diseases.**

Lipoid nephrosis (Epstein's nephrosis)

A disease of the kidneys responsible for the spillage of much protein in the urine. This disorder may be accompanied by swelling of the legs (edema) and increased cholesterol in the blood.
Homeopathy may be effective in treating this ailment; check with your doctor.

Lipoma

These are benign fatty tumors of the skin. They cannot generally be treated by Homeopathy.
Nevertheless, you may try using:
GRAPHITES 5 C,
three pellets, three times a day,
over a period of two months.
If the condition persists, see your doctor.

Lipothymia (Syncope, fainting)

WARNING: You should always see a doctor after any fainting or "blacking out" spell.

Lips

Swollen lips (an allergic swelling of the face and particularly of the lips, due to a disorder of the blood vessels and surrounding nerves):
Depending on symptoms, take three pellets three times a day.
● if the person is not thirsty,
APIS MELLIFICA 9 C.
● if thirsty,
BELLADONNA 9 C.

Cracked lips: (same dosage)
● cracks that are yellow, located at the corner of the mouth,
GRAPHITES 9 C.
● cracks that are red, located at the corner of the mouth,
NITRICUM ACIDUM 9 C.
● lip is cracked vertically in the middle,
NATRUM MURIATICUM 9 C.

Dry lips: (same dosage)
BRYONIA ALBA 9 C,
for the most common cases.
Supplement with:
ARUM TRIPHYLLUM 9 C,
if skin tends to peel off.

▷ *Also see* **Herpes.**

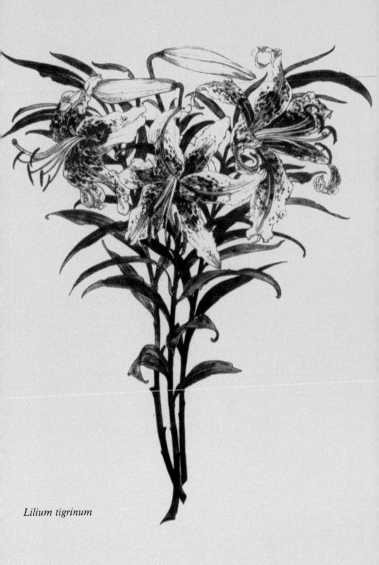

Lilium tigrinum

Lithiasis
(Cholelithiasis, urinary lithiasis)

▷ *See* **Colic, Calculi.**

Liver

If you are suffering from any of the following symptoms, take three pellets of the listed remedy three times a day.

- a sharp pain around the liver,
  BRYONIA ALBA 9 C.
- nausea when pressing over the liver,
  CARDUUS MARIANUS 9 C.
- pain in the liver radiating up to the right shoulder,
  CHELIDONIUM MAJUS 9 C.
- yellowish complexion, jaundice,
  CHELIDONIUM MAJUS 9 C.
- gold-yellow stools that float,
  CHELIDONIUM MAJUS 9 C.
- pain in the region of the liver, which is relieved by rubbing,
  PODOPHYLLUM PELTATUM 9 C.

WARNING: Remember the liver may cause, or be related to, a number of diseases. You should check with your doctor any time you have jaundice, or pain around the liver.

▷ *Also see* **Colic, Diarrhea, Hemorrhoids, Migraines, Nausea, Vertigo, Vomiting.**

Long-term preventive remedy

▷ *See* **Terrain.**

Loosening of the teeth

▷ *See* **Teeth.**

Lordosis (Saddleback)

A concave curving of the spinal column. May be accompanied by back pain.

▷ *See* **Spinal column.**

Loss of balance
(while walking)

▷ *See* **Gait.**

Lumbago

▷ *See* **Spinal column.**

Lump in the throat

- *If you feel there's a lump in your throat when you get upset,* take:
  IGNATIA AMARA 9 C,
  three pellets three times a day.
- *If the sensation of a lump in your throat is made worse by swallowing:*
  LACHESIS 9 C,
  three pellets three times a day.
- *If you feel a lump rising from your stomach to your throat:*
  ASAFOETIDA 9 C,
  three pellets three times a day.

Lungs

▷ *See* **Shortness of Breath, Coughing, Congestion, Pleurisy, Pneumonia.**

Lycopodium clavatum

Base substance: the spores of Club moss.
Suitable for:
Sedentary individuals who have

trouble eliminating waste material; their digestive tracts seem lazy (particularly the liver) but their minds are quick.

Characteristic signs and symptoms:
Repressed anger; the need to have someone near but refusal to speak to them; difficulty in waking up in the morning; slow digestion; red face after eating; drowsiness after meals, made worse by taking a nap; abdominal bloating, particularly in the lower part of the abdomen; a craving for sugar; inability to digest, or aversion to oysters; hemorrhoids; acetone on the breath; red stones passed in the urine; a craving for air; stopped up nose; sore throat beginning with the right tonsil then moving to the left one; sore throat relieved by drinking something warm; marked right-sided location of all symptoms; general worsening of condition around 5 p.m., or early evening.

Main clinical uses:
Nervous or emotional breakdown; gout; face flushing; poor digestion; liver or kidney pain; chronic constipation; hemorrhoids.

WARNING: If condition worsens or persists for more than 72 hours, check with your physician.

Lycopus virginicus

Base substance: Virginia horehound or Bugle weed.

Characteristic signs and symptoms:
Palpitations; weakness of the heart; passing diluted, watery urine; eyes that seem to be popping out of their sockets.

Main clinical uses:
Nervous heart; palpitations; hyperthyroiditis: *WARNING - These diseases are serious. Contact your physician immediately for treatment recommendation.*

Lymphatism
(the Lymphatic temperament)

Sluggishness, a sluggish attitude and action. This is basically a character trait and may not respond to any sort of treatment.
Try:
GELSEMIUM SEMPERVIRENS 9 C, NATRUM MURIATICUM 9 C, alternate three pellets of each, two weeks a month, over a period of three months.

Lymph nodes, Adenitis

The presence of a swollen or inflamed lymph node doesn't constitute a diagnosis in itself.

WARNING: Check with your doctor to find out what has caused it.

In the meantime, take:
MERCURIUS SOLUBILIS 9 C, three pellets three times a day.

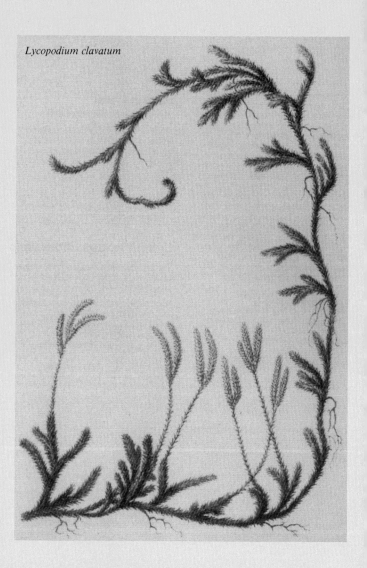

Lycopodium clavatum

MN

*"The extreme smallness
of the doses used in Homeopathy
corresponds to a great number
of facts observed by doctors
throughout the ages and to the soundest
principles of science."*

SEBASTIEN DES GUIDI

Magnesia carbonica

Base substance: Magnesium carbonate.

Characteristic signs and symptoms:
Hyperacidity, particularly of sweat and diarrhea; very greenish stools, like pond water; toothache relieved by walking.

Main clinical uses:
Gastroenteritis; acid dyspepsia; toothache.

Magnesia muriatica

Base substance: Magnesium chloride.

Characteristic signs and symptoms:
Constipation with tiny, marble-sized stools; enlarged liver that is painful to the touch; inability to digest milk.

Main clinical uses:
Constipation.
Hepatic insufficiency: *WARNING - This disease is serious. You should consult your physician for advice.*

Magnesia phosphorica

Base substance: Magnesium phosphate.

Characteristic signs and symptoms:
Spasms; severe crampy abdominal pains, improved by doubling up and applying heat and pressure.

Main clinical uses:
Facial neuralgia; toothache; writer's cramp; abdominal pain or cramps; menstrual period pains; sciatica.

WARNING: If condition worsens or persists for more than 72 hours, check with your physician.

Malaria

Malaria can only be treated with regular, non-homeopathic medicines.

For the lingering effects of malaria (they can last for years) take:
CINCHONA OFFICINALIS 9 C, three pellets, three times a day, twenty days a month, over a period of three months.

Mania

Intense psychic arousal, abnormal exhilaration. This may indicate a behavioral disorder and should be talked about with a doctor.
True mania is not within the realm of Homeopathy, but is instead within that of psychiatry.

Manic depression

Alternation of mania and depression.
See a psychiatrist or speak to your regular family doctor.

Manufacturing of Homeopathic Medicines (The)

▷ *See* **Homeopathic medicines.**

Mastoiditis

Consult your homeopathic physician.

Mastosis

▷ *See* **Breasts.**

Masturbation

▷ *See* **Sexual Disorders.**

Materia Medica

The *Materia Medica* is a book that the homeopathic physician studies to learn the action of various homeopathic medicines he or she will use in practice. The study of a particular remedy is known as a *"proving."*
Provings include the study of three types of symptoms:
- symptoms observed after experimentation with the substance in question on healthy individuals (see **Homeopathic theory**),
- symptoms observed after accidental or intentional medicinal intoxication,
- symptoms observed by homeopathic physicians and cured by the administering of a remedy, unknown to do so in the original experiments.

Measles

What you suspect to be measles should be seen by a doctor.
For diagnosed measles, you may give your child:
BELLADONNA 9 C,
MORBILLINUM NOSODE 9 C,
SULPHUR 9 C,
alternate three pellets of each, three times a day.

Medicinal aggravation

At the beginning of a homeopathic treatment, the patient often has the impression that the symptoms have intensified and that former symptoms have come back. This "aggravation" is usually quite bearable and is most often compatible with normal daily activities.
Medicinal aggravation is a good sign, for it means that the treatment was correctly chosen and the body is indeed reacting. After a few days, symptoms will decrease and finally disappear. The point of cure is then reached.
If the person feels that this temporary aggravation is too unpleasant, the treatment may be halted for a few days and taken up once more later. When the treatment is resumed, "aggravation" should not recur.
If you experience medicinal aggravation, try not to think "Homeopathy isn't right for me" but stick with it. The reaction you are feeling is a sign that the medicine is working and a cure can be expected. Medicinal aggravation should rarely be encountered if you follow the therapeutic advice in this *Guide*. It may occur more often in the course of a terrain treatment to cure a chronic illness (see **Terrain**).

Medicine cabinet

Which 35 homeopathic remedies should you keep in your family medicine cabinet?

▷ *See* **Family Kit.**

Melancholy

The symptoms of melancholy (apathy, indifference, mental sluggishness, depression) may be treated by Homeopathy but only under the strict guidance of a homeopathic physician. Melancholy can be a serious mental disorder with guilt complex, self-accusation, and risk of suicide. See your doctor.

Melilotus officinalis

Base substance: Melilot or sweet clover.

Characteristic signs and symptoms:
Migraine headache with red face;
symptoms are relieved when nose
bleeds.

Main clinical uses: Migraines; nosebleed.

Memory

Good memory is often a question of
good attention. If you've become too
busy to pay attention to the world
around you (to others and to yourself
and your body), you might find it
harder to remember things. Try to use
your eyes and ears to develop visual
and auditory memory as much or
more than just "plain memory."
Trying to visualize or hear things
again will help you to sharpen and
maintain your memory.

As a supplementary aid, take three
pellets of one of the following
remedies three times a day:

*Depending on why there seems to be a
memory loss:*
- for aging (older people may find it
harder to remember than before),
BARYTA CARBONICA 9 C.
- mild learning disabilities of children,
BARYTA CARBONICA 9 C.
- if you seem slow to understand or
grasp a concept,
CONIUM MACULATUM 9 C.
- mental strain,
KALI PHOSPHORICUM 9 C.
- apathy and indifference,
PHOSPHORICUM ACIDUM 9 C.

Depending on what you forget:
- names,
ANACARDIUM ORIENTALE 9 C.
- your way around the neighborhood,
BARYTA CARBONICA 9 C.
- your train of thought or what you're
supposed to be doing,
CALADIUM SEGUINUM 9 C.
- mixing up words and sentences,
LYCOPODIUM CLAVATUM 9 C.
- recent events,
SULPHUR 9 C.

Ménière's disease

*WARNING: See a doctor or
neurologist.*

An affection characterized by extreme
dizziness often accompanied by
buzzing in the ears, nausea and
deafness.

Menopause

Menopause does not necessarily need
to be treated with hormone
replacement therapy. See your
homeopathic doctor. The following
suggestions may help during
menopause.

Take three pellets of the appropriate
remedy three times a day:

Restlessness,
LACHESIS 9 C.

Need of air,
SULPHUR 9 C.

Hot flashes:
- hot flashes made worse at onset of
menstrual flow,
CIMICIFUGA RACEMOSA 9 C.
- hot flashes improved at onset of
menstrual flow,
LACHESIS 9 C.

Mental strain,
SEPIA 9 C.

General fatigue,
CINCHONA OFFICINALIS 9 C.

Bleeding: (See your doctor.)
LACHESIS 9 C.

Hemorrhoids,
LACHESIS 9 C.

*Aversion to tight-fitting clothes,
necklaces, scarves around the neck,*
LACHESIS 9 C.

Red cheeks,
SANGUINARIA CANADENSIS 9 C.

Migraines,
SANGUINARIA CANADENSIS 9 C.

Rheumatism, joint pains,
  CIMICIFUGA RACEMOSA 9 C.

Nosebleeds,
  LACHESIS 9 C.

Sadness,
  SEPIA 9 C.

Talkativeness,
  LACHESIS 9 C.

If you have other symptoms, look them up under the appropriate headings and eventually consult a doctor or gynecologist.

Menstrual periods

Depending on symptoms, alternate three pellets of one or more of the following remedies three times daily:

Unusually heavy periods:
* heavy periods and fatigue,
  CINCHONA OFFICINALIS 9 C.
  HELONIAS DIOICA 9 C.
* heavy periods with black or dark blood,
  CROCUS SATIVUS 9 C.
* painful heavy flow when moving,
  ERIGERON CANADENSE 9 C.

Missed periods or "amenorrhea":
* missing periods after being frightened,
  ACONITUM NAPELLUS 9 C.
* after catching cold,
  ACONITUM NAPELLUS 9 C.
* after being angry,
  COLOCYNTHIS 9 C.
* after mental strain,
  NATRUM MURIATICUM 9 C.
* after getting wet,
  PULSATILLA 9 C.
* without cause and when bleeding occurs in another organ at the time a menstrual period is due (for example, a nosebleed),
  SENECIO AUREUS 9 C.

Early periods:
* early periods with clots of blood,
  BELLADONNA 9 C.
* every time things go wrong,
  CALCAREA CARBONICA 9 C.

* early periods with dark blood,
  CYCLAMEN EUROPAEUM 9 C.
* early periods with red blood,
  SABINA 9 C.

Pre-period symptoms:
* general bloated feeling with anxiety and "pickiness," or desire to straighten up the house,
  SEPIA 9 C.

▷ *Also see* **Premenstrual Syndrome.**

Painful periods or "dysmenorrhea":
* painful periods with a sensation of heaviness in the lower pelvic region,
  BELLADONNA 9 C.
* pain aggravated by being moved or jolted (during a car ride, for example),
  BELLADONNA 9 C.
* pain in the right ovary,
  BELLADONNA 9 C.
* pain radiating in all directions,
  CAULOPHYLLUM THALICTROIDES 9 C.
* intolerable pain,
  CHAMOMILLA 9 C.
* pain in the left ovary,
  LACHESIS 9 C.
* pain occurring just when menstrual flow stops (pain stops if flow starts up again),
  LACHESIS 9 C.
* pain in the thighs, the sacrum, or the pubic bone,
  SABINA 9 C.
* pain in the back,
  SENECIO AUREUS 9 C.
* pain with cold sweating,
  VERATRUM ALBUM 9 C.

Very light periods:
* flow is light or stops and then starts again,
  PULSATILLA 9 C.
* fewer days of flow than usual,
  SEPIA 9 C.

General symptoms during menstrual periods:
See the heading corresponding to the actual symptoms.

Late periods:
* until they come, take:
  PULSATILLA 9 C.

Bleeding between periods:
   CINCHONA OFFICINALIS 5 C.
   (If this happens, check with a
   doctor.)

▷ *See* **Ovulation.**

If you're taking a homeopathic
treatment, there is no need to stop it
during your period unless indicated by
your doctor. Check with your doctor
or gynecologist if you have any
concern about unusual bleeding or
periods.

▷ *Also see* **Menopause, Puberty.**

Mental confusion

*Anyone who finds it hard to think
clearly* may try:
   BARYTA CARBONICA 9 C,
   three pellets three times a day.
   This treatment may be continued
   indefinitely.

*WARNING: Check with your doctor if
mental confusion follows head injury,
or if it persists. Any head injury should
be reported to your doctor immediately.*

Menyanthes trifoliata

Base substance: Marsh trefoil or Water
shamrock.

Main clinical use:
Migraine with an ice-cold feeling,
particularly in the feet.

Mercurius corrosivus

Base substance: Corrosive sublimate of
mercury.

Characteristic signs and symptoms:
Ulceration of the mucous membranes;
constant need to pass stools but feeling
unrelieved by defecating; constant
need to urinate; inflammation of the
eye; purulent sore throat and mouth;
inflammation of the urethra.

Main clinical uses:
Inflammation of the colon; purulent
conjunctivitis: *WARNING - These
diseases are serious. Contact your
physician immediately for treatment
recommendation.*
Dysentery; cystitis; aphthae; purulent
sore throat.

Mercurius solubilis Hahnemanni

Base substance: "Soluble" mercury
prepared according to a special
method devised by Hahnemann.

Characteristic signs and symptoms:
Bad breath; tongue that retains teeth
marks; excess salivation (the patient
drools on pillow); bleeding gums; sore
throat covered with white spots;
diarrhea; tendency toward purulent
ulceration; swollen lymph nodes;
nocturnal sweating; fever occurring at
night accompanied by shivering;
prolonged fever; trembling of the
hands.

Main clinical uses:
Sore throat; aphthae; pharyngitis;
pyorrhea; rectal inflammation.

*WARNING: If condition worsens or
persists for more than 72 hours, check
with your physician.*

Metritis

▷ *See* **Uterus.**

Mezereum

Base substance: Spurge olive.

Characteristic signs and symptoms:
Cutaneous vesicles developing with
white crusts and surrounding
ulcerations; intense itching, worse at
night; neuralgia; alternation of skin
eruptions and internal disorders.

Main clinical uses:
Eczema; impetigo.
Herpes zoster (shingles); neuralgia
following herpes zoster; facial
neuralgia: *WARNING - These diseases
are serious. Contact your physician
immediately for treatment
recommendation.*

Microbial infection

Homeopathic medicine will reinforce
the body's defense mechanisms,
helping it to get rid of pathogenic
bacteria. You must see your doctor.
Homeopathic medicines taken early
may be helpful, but you may require
antibiotics.

Micturition (Disorders of)

▷ *See* **Urinating (Difficulty in).**

Migraines

Treating migraine headaches:
Migraines are deep-seated pains
affecting half the head. It's believed
that these particularly painful
headaches occur from a swelling of the
vessels inside the head. Their cause is
not clearly understood.

Certain types of migraines may
respond to the following remedies.
Take three pellets every half hour *as
soon as symptoms occur.* If you do this
in time, you stand a better chance of
success even if you also take a
non-homeopathic medicine for the
headache.
- for a throbbing migraine,
  BELLADONNA 9 C.
- migraine with a sensation of heat in
  the head and cold in the extremities,
  CARBO VEGETABILIS 9 C.
- migraine in the back of the head,
  heavy eyelids, and the passing of large
  amounts of colorless urine,
  GELSEMIUM SEMPERVIRENS 9 C.
- ophthalmic migraine,
  IRIS VERSICOLOR 9 C.
- migraine with bilious vomiting and
  burning in the stomach,
  IRIS VERSICOLOR 9 C.
- migraine with bilious diarrhea,
  NATRUM SULPHURICUM 9 C.
- migraine preceded by intense hunger
  or a feeling of well-being,
  PSORINUM 9 C.
- migraine with burping,
  SANGUINARIA CANADENSIS 9 C.
- migraine with red cheeks,
  particularly the right cheek,
  SANGUINARIA CANADENSIS 9 C.

*WARNING: If symptoms persist,
discontinue use of the above remedies
and consult your physician.*

▷ *Also see* **Headache.** Although
migraines and headaches may be
clinically different, they sometimes
respond to the same remedies.

Long-term preventive treatment:
If a homeopathic treatment for an
acute migraine headache fails, talk to a
homeopathic physician. It may be
possible to find a long-term treatment
that helps prevent or decrease the
number of migraine headaches you
suffer from.

Milk

▷ *See* **Breast-feeding.**

For milk in the breasts of a
non-pregnant woman:
    PULSATILLA 9 C,
      three pellets three times a day.

Millefolium

Base substance: Yarrow.

Main clinical use: Bleeding of bright
red blood.

Mint

Why shouldn't mint be used during a
homeopathic treatment?

▷ *See* **Antidotes.**

Miscarriage, spontaneous abortion
(Tendency to)

If the patient has a tendency to abort
spontaneously (miscarriage), she
should take the following (as well as
seek the advice of her doctor or
midwife):
    SABINA 9 C,
      three pellets three times a day
      throughout the pregnancy.

Morphology

▷ *See* **Typology.**

Moschus

Base substance: Musk.

Characteristic signs and symptoms:
Fainting with excessive pretentions of
suffering; uncontrollable laughter;

quarrelsome moods; various types of
spasms.

Main clinical uses:
Mental strain or nervous outbreaks.
Fainting spells: *WARNING - Any
fainting spell must be told to your
doctor to determine the exact nature of
its cause.*

Mosquito bites

▷ *See* **Insect bites.**

Mother-tincture

The mother-tincture is the base
preparation of homeopathic products
whenever they are of animal or
vegetable origin.
The plant or animal product is placed
in a mixture of water and alcohol and
macerated. **Dilution** and **potentization**
(see these entries), which are essential
to the preparation of the **homeopathic
medicine,** are then carried out under
careful laboratory control. The
mother-tincture (usually abbreviated,
"M.T.") contains a measurable dose of
the base substance, so caution must be
exercised to avoid possible toxic
effects when handling this type of
product (see **Danger in Homeopathy**).

*WARNING: In this text, many base
substances are mentioned and are
available in tincture form, some of
which could be very dangerous (Nux
Vomica, Aconite) but exist as a
medical necessity to prepare
homeopathic dilutions.*

Mouth

Take three pellets three times a day of
one or several of the following
medicines.

Thrush (yeast infections, candida) of the mouth: *WARNING - This disease is serious. Contact your physician immediately for treatment recommendation.*

Your doctor may prescribe as follows:
- thrush sores with a burning sensation in the mouth, relieved by warmth,
  ARSENICUM ALBUM 9 C.
- thrush sores that bleed when touched,
  BORAX 9 C.
- painful thrush sores when touched by food (especially in children),
  BORAX 9 C.
- thrush with much saliva and bad breath,
  MERCURIUS SOLUBILIS 9 C.
- thrush with sharp pains around the sores,
  NITRICUM ACIDUM 9 C.
- thrush sores with oozing, yellow pus,
  SULPHURICUM ACIDUM 9 C.

A further treatment for all of the above is to swab a small amount of PLANTAGO MAJOR M.T., diluted in boiled lukewarm water, to the affected area.

Teeth: ▷ *see* this entry.

Gums (gingivitis):
- if the gums are swollen and spongy,
  MERCURIUS SOLUBILIS 9 C.
- for bleeding gums,
  PHOSPHORUS 9 C.

Taste problems:
- if you have the taste of rotten eggs in your mouth,
  ARNICA MONTANA 9 C.
- if your usual coffee suddenly tastes bad,
  IGNATIA AMARA 9 C.
- if you have a salty or metallic taste in your mouth,
  MERCURIUS SOLUBILIS 9 C.

- if you have a bad taste in your mouth that you can't really describe, or a clay-like taste, or no taste at all (as during a cold, for example),
  PULSATILLA 9 C.
- if you have an acid taste in the mouth,
  NUX VOMICA 9 C.

Breath: ▷ *see* this entry.

Herpes: ▷ *see* this entry.

Tongue: ▷ *see* this entry.

Lips: ▷ *see* this entry.

Pyorrhea: ▷ *see* **Teeth.**

Stomatitis (inflammation of the mouth):
  BORAX 9 C.
  MERCURIUS SOLUBILIS 9 C,
  alternate three pellets of each.

Multiple sclerosis

This disease cannot be treated by Homeopathy. See your regular doctor or a neurologist.

Mumps

WARNING: Check with your doctor.

Inflammation of the parotid glands which are located in the cheeks.
If a doctor has already diagnosed this self-limiting disease, he or she may prescribe:
  MERCURIUS SOLUBILIS 9 C,
  PULSATILLA 9 C,
  SULPHUR 9 C,
  alternate three pellets of each, three times a day for ten days.

To help prevent adults from catching mumps (males run a risk of sterility from testicular inflammation), avoid contact and take:
  TRIFOLIUM REPENS 3 X,
  ten drops, three times a day for ten days.

Muscles

Muscle strain: (sharp stabbing pain in a muscle)
ARNICA MONTANA 9 C,
three pellets three times a day.

Muscular contracture or spasms:
MAGNESIA PHOSPHORICA 9 C,
three pellets three times a day.

▷ *See* **Spasms.**

Stiffness, soreness:
▷ *see* **Stiffness.**

Cramps: ▷ *see* this entry.

Muscle pains:
RHUS TOXICODENDRON 9 C,
three pellets three times a day.

Mycosis (Dermatomycosis)

WARNING: Consult your doctor.
Skin disease caused by the presence of fungi.
Take:
ARSENICUM IODATUM 5 C,
SEPIA 5 C,
alternate three pellets of each,
three times a day.
CALENDULA M.T. may be applied to
the affected areas twice a day.

Myelitis

This term refers to various inflammatory diseases of the spinal cord, none of which can be treated by Homeopathy. See your regular doctor or neurologist.

Myxedema

▷ See **Thyroid gland.**

Nails

The condition of your nails is often a good reflection of what is going on inside your body: if your nails don't look normal, you may benefit from a homeopathic treatment. Do not count on local treatments to fortify them. Instead, take three pellets of one of the following remedies three times a day over a period of three months.

• for cracked, deformed or split nails, or for nails that don't grow,
ANTIMONIUM CRUDUM 9 C.

• for brittle nails, nails that break, nails under which the skin is inflamed, overly thick nails,
GRAPHITES 9 C.

• for abnormally raised, rounded nails,
NITRICUM ACIDUM 9 C.

• for ridges running the length of the nails or white spots on the nails,
SILICEA 9 C.

• for ingrown nails (take the following remedy after a visit to your doctor or podiatrist; it will help prevent relapses),
TEUCRIUM MARUM VERUM 9 C.

• for soft nails or nails with wavy ridges across them,
THUJA OCCIDENTALIS 9 C.

Naja tripudians

Base substance: Cobra venom.

Characteristic signs and symptoms:
Heart murmur due to lesions of the valves; palpitations which make it difficult for the patient to speak; pain

in the region of the heart; weak heart; hypotension.

Main clinical uses:
Palpitations; angina pectoris; weak heart; tonic for patients with heart disease: *WARNING - These diseases are extremely serious. Contact your physician immediately for treatment recommendation.*

Naphthalinum

Base substance: Naphthaline.

Main clinical use:
This remedy slows down the evolution of eye disease lesions (cataract, opacity of the cornea).

WARNING: An eye doctor must be consulted.

Natrum carbonicum

Base substance: Sodium carbonate.

Suitable for: The chronic aftereffects of sunstroke.

Characteristic signs and symptoms:
Depression aggravated by mental strain or the summer heat; generalized edema; headache after being exposed to the sun; chronic or repeated pains.

Main clinical uses:
The aftereffects of sunstroke; mental strain or breakdown; sprains.

Natrum muriaticum

Base substance: Sodium chloride, or table salt.

Suitable for:
People who are thin, especially the upper half of their bodies, although they eat well; these people also have oily perspiration, and are often reserved, uncommunicative and absent-minded.

Characteristic signs and symptoms:
Sadness; depression; condition made worse when in the presence of other people, or when consoled in an untactful way; person mulls over his problems; craving for salt; intense thirst; dryness of the mucous membranes; "map-like tongue"; repeated allergic colds; herpes; rashes occurring at the edge of the hair line; headaches with visual loss; pain in the lumbar region, relieved by lying on a hard surface; condition worse near the sea or during exposure to the sun.

Main clinical uses:
Ophthalmic migraines; spasmodic coryza; hay fever; sinusitis; allergy to sunlight; eczema; herpes; aphthosis; anemia; Grave's disease; spasmophilia; mental strain or breakdown.

Natrum sulphuricum

Base substance: Sodium sulfate.

Suitable for: Symptoms of head trauma.

Characteristic signs and symptoms:
Behavioral changes (increased sensitivity) following trauma to the head; music causes aggravation; migraines; bilious diarrhea after breakfast; asthma due to a change in the weather; general aggravation by exposure to humidity; eczema, with large yellowish scales; itching when getting undressed.

Main clinical uses:
Syndromes after head trauma: *WARNING - Contact your physician immediately for treatment recommendation. (Head trauma demands a medical and neurological examination).*
Mental strain or breakdown; migraine; diarrhea; asthma; rheumatism; eczema.

Natural medicine
(General Principles of)

Homeopathy is based on the **reactional** capabilities of the human body. You may treat your ailment by Homeopathy and respect the principle of natural medicine: avoiding useless aggressions to your body. You can start by avoiding, or at least limiting, the use of some of these now: deodorants, birth control pills, cortisone ointments, and unnecessary surgical removal of hemorrhoids or varicose veins (see these topics). A medical doctor also trained in Homeopathy can help you decide when certain medicines and surgery might be necessary.

Nausea

If you should suffer from nausea, take three pellets of one of the following remedies every hour or three times a day.

Depending on the cause:
- following an operation on the abdomen,
  BISMUTHUM METALLICUM 9 C.
- after catching a chill,
  COCCULUS INDICUS 9 C.
- motion sickness or when watching things move by (telephone poles, stripes on a highway, etc.),
  COCCULUS INDICUS 9 C.
- when looking at, smelling or thinking about food,
  COLCHICUM AUTUMNALE 9 C.
- after an episode of coughing,
  IPECAC 9 C.
- after meals,
  NUX VOMICA 9 C.
- while smoking,
  NUX VOMICA 9 C.
- during menstrual periods,
  NUX VOMICA 9 C.

- during pregnancy,
  SEPIA 9 C.

Depending on the circumstances:
- nausea relieved by drinking liquids,
  BRYONIA ALBA 9 C.
- nausea relieved by eating,
  SEPIA 9 C.

Depending on the accompanying symptoms:
- nausea with dizziness,
  COCCULUS INDICUS 9 C.
- with uncoated tongue and much saliva,
  IPECAC 9 C.

Neck pains

▷ *See* **Rheumatism.**

After choosing the appropriate treatment from the list under this heading, supplement it with the following:
  LACHNANTHES TINCTORIA 9 C,
  three pellets three times a day.

Nephritis
(Inflammation of the kidneys)

Certain cases of acute nephritis (inflammation of the kidney often accompanied by swelling of the ankles and passing protein in the urine) may be treated by Homeopathy. Check with a homeopathic physician.

Nephrocolic
(Renal colic, Kidney stones)

▷ *See* **Colic.**

Nervous agitation

▷ *See* below, **Nervousness.**

Nervousness

We all become nervous at times, but this is not always bad. Our innate capacity to react mentally and emotionally to the world around us is sometimes an instinctive response to trouble, and a way of protecting ourselves. Let's say, then, that nervousness in proper measure is a good thing.

Abnormal nervousness begins when people over-react, or when they stay nervous and wrought after a trying time has passed and they should have returned to a normal, daily routine of living. When anxiety and nervousness master the individual, rather than the other way around, they've become pathological. Your nervousness then needs to be talked over with your doctor.

A homeopathic physician might make a good person to listen to you; he or she will then in turn ask you several questions concerning your mental and emotional functioning in the course of your everyday life (your homeopath may ask you about your mental and emotional health even if you came because of a "simple" physical ailment. The mind has an important influence on the body's health, so it is normal for your homeopathic doctor to try and understand your health problems in the context of your total personality).

To better understand how to treat mild, short-term anxiety states, *see* **Anxiety, Depression, Emotion, Children, Neurosis.**

Nervousness before an event

Take three pellets of one of the following remedies three times a day.

During exam periods, begin the night before.

ARGENTUM NITRICUM 9 C,
if the nervousness speeds up your thought processes and makes you feel like you have to get everything over with before you begin.

GELSEMIUM SEMPERVIRENS 9 C,
if your mind seems slowed down, giving the impression of exhaustion.

Both remedies may also work for decreasing diarrhea before stressful events or examinations.

▷ *See* **Anxiety.**

Neuralgia

Pain in a nerve ending. Usually, a sharp pain running the length of a nerve. Homeopathic medicines may help relieve the pains. Take three pellets of one or more of the following remedies three times a day or every hour.

Depending on the cause of the neuralgia:
- dry cold,
  ACONITUM NAPELLUS 9 C.
- damp weather,
  DULCAMARA 9 C.
- trauma to a nerve,
  HYPERICUM PERFORATUM 9 C.
- herpes zoster—shingles, (Check with your doctor first.)
  MEZEREUM 9 C.

Depending on the modifying circumstances:
Aggravated by:
- drafts of air,
  CINCHONA OFFICINALIS 9 C.
- night air,
  MEZEREUM 9 C.
- stormy weather,
  RHODODENDRON CHRYSANTHEMUM 9 C.

Improved by:
- pressure, heat, or by doubling up,
  MAGNESIA PHOSPHORICA 9 C.

Depending on the accompanying sensations:
- numbness,
  ACONITUM NAPELLUS 9 C.
- throbbing,
  BELLADONNA 9 C.
- the path of pain feels very narrow, like a thread,
  COFFEA CRUDA 9 C.
- pain moves along the nerve,
  COLOCYNTHIS 9 C.
- shooting pains,
  KALMIA LATIFOLIA 9 C.
- sudden, violent pains,
  MAGNESIA PHOSPHORICA 9 C.
- pains that feel like electric shocks,
  PHYTOLACCA DECANDRA 9 C.
- urge to move legs although no real pain is felt,
  ZINCUM METALLICUM 9 C.

▷ As needed, *look up* the following: **Face, Intercostal pain, Sciatica, Teeth.**

Neurasthenia

Nervous exhaustion, marked by irritability and weakness.

▷ See **Depression.**

Neuritis

▷ See **Neuralgia.**

Neurosis

A condition of tension or irritability of the nervous system, which is based on no evident cause. The person's behavior may seem unbearable but he or she is not lost touch with reality. Neurosis should not be confused with **psychosis** which defines severe

emotional illness where the patient is out of touch with reality (insanity). Many normally functioning people have neuroses; the awareness of having a neurosis is a precondition to treating it successfully with **psychotherapy** (see this heading). You must want to get over a neurosis for psychotherapy to work.
You may prepare for such a treatment by Homeopathy, preferably a homeopathic treatment devised by you and a homeopathic physician. You may, however, start with one of the following medicines at a rate of three pellets three times a day.
- for physical symptoms from a neurosis (feeling of oppression, lump in the throat, etc.),
  IGNATIA AMARA 9 C.
- for constant mulling over of ideas, repeated corrections of one's actions, obsession,
  NATRUM MURIATICUM 9 C.
- for irrational anxiety with a need for company and the fear of becoming seriously ill,
  PHOSPHORUS 9 C.

▷ For fear or "phobia," *see* **Fear.**

Nevus

A nevus is any congenital lesion (mole, bump, etc.) or discolored patch (birthmark, spot, freckle, etc.) of the skin caused by pigmentation or increased formation of blood vessels. There is no corresponding homeopathic treatment.

Don't have a nevus (plural: nevi) removed unless:
- it is constantly irritated by an external contact with shirt collars, bra straps, or while shaving, etc.
- its appearance changes (color, shape, thickness),

- or unless your doctor advises its removal.

In this case, take:
PHOSPHORUS 5 C,
THUJA OCCIDENTALIS 5 C,
alternate three pellets of each, three times a day for a period of two weeks following the operation.

▷ For vascular nevus or "port wine stains," see **Angioma.**

Nightmares

A child who has nightmares and cries in his or her sleep may be given:
STRAMONIUM 9 C,
three pellets when the child starts having bad dreams or crying, if this happens only occasionally. If it occurs more regularly, give the same amount every night at bedtime.

Nitricum acidum

Base substance: Nitric acid.

Suitable for:
Irritable people who can't stand sympathy and understanding.

Characteristic signs and symptoms:
Cracks at the junctions of skin and mucous membranes with a prickly sensation and bleeding; warts surrounded by yellow skin with sharp pain on pressure; burning, foul-smelling pus; skin ulcerations.

Main clinical uses:
Fissural eczema; anal cracking; fever blisters; cold sores; warts; leg ulcers.

Noise (Intolerance to)

IGNATIA AMARA 9 C,
three pellets three times a day.

Nose

For problems of the nose, take three pellets of one of the following remedies three times a day.

Stopped-up nose,
NUX VOMICA 9 C.
Crusts inside the nose,
KALI BICHROMICUM 9 C.
Itchy nose,
CINA 9 C.
Sneezing,
NUX VOMICA 9 C.
Cracks on the edge of a nostril,
NITRICUM ACIDUM 9 C.
Boils,
HEPAR SULPHURIS CALCAREUM 9 C.
Sense of smell:
• overly sensitive nose to the smell of food,
COLCHICUM AUTUMNALE 9 C.
• to the smell of tobacco, coffee, perfume,
IGNATIA AMARA 9 C.
• to the smell of flowers,
SABADILLA 9 C.
• everything seems to have a bad smell,
SULPHUR 9 C.
• loss of the sense of smell (anosmia, olfactory anesthesia),
KALI BICHROMICUM 9 C.

Colds:
▷ see this entry.

Hay fever:
▷ see this entry.

Redness of the nose,
CARBO ANIMALIS 9 C.

Nosebleeding:
▷ see **Bleeding.**

Sinusitis:
▷ see this entry.

Ulceration or excoriation inside the nose:
KALI BICHROMICUM 5 C.

Nosebleeds

▷ *See* **Bleeding.**

Numbness (Feeling of)

If one of your extremities (arm or leg)
feels numb, take:
COCCULUS INDICUS 9 C,
three pellets, once an hour.
Consult a homeopathic physician if
the problem persists.

▷ *Also see* **Hyperventilation.**

Nux moschata

Base substance: Nutmeg.

Characteristic signs and symptoms:
Irresistible drowsiness; a tendency to
faint; moodiness; marked dryness of
the mucous membranes, particularly
the mouth (without thirst); saliva feels
like cotton; abdominal bloating.

Main clinical uses:
Drowsiness; dyspepsia due to flatulence.

Nux vomica

Base substance: Poison nut.

Suitable for:
Irritable, sedentary people who
overwork their digestive tracts with
large amounts of coffee and tobacco.

Characteristic signs and symptoms:
Sensitivity to all kinds of external
stimulus (noise, light, smells, cold);
frequent sneezing attacks in the
morning; congested nose at night and
runny nose during the day; digestive
spasms of the gut; stomachache after
meals; drowsiness after meals that is
relieved by a short nap; constipation
without being able to go; internal
hemorrhoids; muscle cramps.

Main clinical uses:
Indigestion and uneasiness brought on
by excessive drinking and/or heavy
meals; spastic dyspepsia; gastritis;
constipation; hemorrhoids; migraines
and poor digestion; gout; lumbago;
coryza; hay fever.

*WARNING: If condition worsens or
persists for more than 72 hours, check
with your physician.*

Nymphomania

▷ *See* **Sexual disorders.**

*"Similars
act upon similars
likewise similars
require similars."*

DEMOCRITES

O P
Q

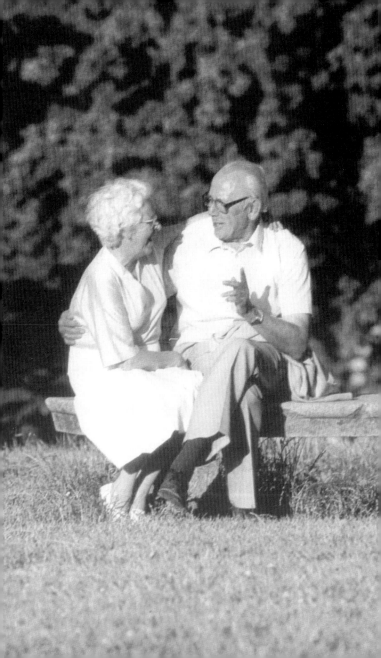

Obsessions

▷ *See* **Neurosis.**

Ointments

The best ointments act on a local skin lesion (sore, blemish, etc.) without affecting the surrounding or underlying tissues (and without being inadvertently absorbed into deeper layers of the body and causing systemic manifestations, such as setting off an attack of asthma).
To treat some skin infections it may be necessary to use an antibiotic cream, but for the majority of minor skin lesions an ointment prepared from CALENDULA will be sufficient to promote healing.
Parasitic infestations of the skin (lice, crabs, mange, etc.) will necessitate the use of a topical medicine prescribed by your doctor.

Old age

Minor, non-specific problems and complaints of aging may be treated, within reasonable limits, with:
BARYTA CARBONICA 9 C,
LACHESIS 5 C,
alternate three pellets of each, three times a day for two weeks a month over a period of several years.
Considering that the elderly often suffer from organic ailments, consult your doctor to handle specific problems and to see whether Homeopathy should be the principal treatment or only an adjunct therapy (for minor disorders).

Operations

▷ *See* **Surgery.**

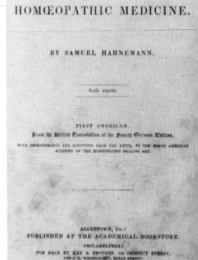

Orchitis

▷ *See* **Testicles.**

Organic diseases

Organic diseases cannot generally be treated by Homeopathy except to slow down their progression, or to relieve some of their symptoms (pain, for example). They are the opposite of **functional diseases** (see this entry).

Organon

The Organon of the Art of Healing is the first book written by Samuel Hahnemann (see **History of**

Homeopathy), the founder of Homeopathy. It was published in Germany in 1810; the first American edition appeared in 1836.

The initial paragraph of the *Organon* stipulates that "the physician's first and only vocation is to reestablish the health of the sick; this is what is meant by the 'Art of Healing'." The fact that Hahnemann spoke of the patient before explaining his method is significant: it indicates that the goal of Homeopathy is to cure rather than engage in intellectual speculation. Hahnemann was a humanist.

Otitis

WARNING: This disease must be treated by a physician.

Inflammation of the ear.

Acute otitis:
BELLADONNA 9 C,
CAPSICUM ANNUUM 9 C,
FERRUM PHOSPHORICUM 9 C,
alternate three pellets of each,
every hour.

WARNING: If there's no improvement within a few hours, discontinue the use of the above remedies and see your doctor.

Recurring otitis:
check with a homeopathic physician. A long-term preventive treatment may be prescribed.

Chronic otitis may cause damage to the eardrum. You need to consult a doctor for a long-term treatment.

Ovaries

For pain:
APIS MELLIFICA 9 C,
BELLADONNA 9 C,
alternate three pellets of each,
three times a day until you can see a doctor or gynecologist.

Cysts: ▷ *see* this entry.

Overwork

Try to avoid the trap of chronic overwork; people who are addicted to work ("workaholics") never want to stop. They may not feel tired but they're really running on nervous energy—not good sense. Take care of your health and slow down.

The first few days will be hard, but after a while you can get back on a normal schedule of rest and work, particularly if you take:

For physical overwork,
ARNICA MONTANA 9 C,
RHUS TOXICODENDRON 9 C,
alternate three pellets of each,
three times a day.

For mental overwork,
KALI PHOSPHORICUM 9 C,
three pellets three times a day.

Ovulation

For abdominal pains or cramps when ovulation occurs, take:
COLOCYNTHIS 9 C,
SABINA 9 C,
alternate three pellets of each,
three times in the same day.

Oxyuris

▷ *See* **Worms (Intestinal).**

Paeonia officinalis

Base substance: the Peony
Main clinical use: Hemorrhoids with anal fissures.

Pain

Some types of pain may be relieved by a homeopathic treatment if the remedy is correctly selected. There is no specific homeopathic "anti-pain" remedy.
What works will depend on the cause, the sensations, the accompanying symptoms, and what makes the pain better or worse, etc. For acute pains, look up the entry concerning the site or location of the pain, or the type of disease causing it.

Paleness

▷ *See* **Anemia.**

Palpitations (Cardioneurosis)

A sudden unpleasant awareness of the heart beat (rhythm may be regular or irregular) due to nervousness. Consult your doctor.

Parasites

Whatever parasitic disease you are suffering from (fungus, yeast, worms, tropical disease, etc.), you will probably need a double treatment: a regular one to kill the parasite and a homeopathic one to modify the terrain and prevent the parasite from coming back. Check with a doctor.

Parathyroid glands

Organic disorders of the parathyroid glands affect mainly calcium and phosphorus metabolism and may require surgery. When the disorder is of a functional nature, Homeopathy may be used to treat it. Check with your doctor.

▷ *See* **Organic Diseases, Functional Diseases.**

Pareira brava

Base substance: Chondodendron tomentosum.
Characteristic signs and symptoms: Cystitis with constant desire to urinate; difficult or impossible urination; the person may even try so hard to urinate as to get down on all fours; enlarged prostate.
Main clinical uses: Cystitis; enlarged prostate; kidney stones: *WARNING - These diseases are serious. Contact your physician immediately for treatment recommendation.*

Paris quadrifolia

Base substance: Four-leaved grass, or Fox grape.
Characteristic signs and symptoms: A sensation that the eyes are being pulled inward; a sensation of a heavy weight on the back of the neck; a sensation of the scalp being drawn tight; neuralgia.
Main clinical uses: Headache; migraines; neuralgia.

Parkinson's disease

A neurological disease of organic origin that cannot be treated by Homeopathy. Symptoms include muscle trembling, "pill-rolling" movements of the hand and muscular rigidity. See your doctor.

▷ *See* **Organic Diseases.**

Parodontosis

▷ *See* **Teeth.**

Parotid gland

▷ *See* **Mumps.**

For other diseases of the parotid glands, check with your doctor.

Pathogenesis

▷ *See* **Materia Medica.**

Pellets

Pharmaceutical pellets are one form in which homeopathic medicines are prescribed. Pellets come in two sizes: granules #20 and globules #35. Granules, which are taken all at once, are packaged in unit-dose tubes; globules are packaged in multi-dose tubes and are generally taken three at a time. For convenience sake, globules #35 are called "pellets" throughout *The Guide.*

Periarthritis

Inflammation of the tendons and parts around a joint, often affecting the shoulder joint.

▷ *See* **Shoulder.**

Period pains
(Painful menstrual cramps)

▷ *See* **Menstrual periods.**

Periphlebitis

▷ *See* **Phlebitis.**

Perleche

Inflammation of the corner of the mouth.

General treatment:
> GRAPHITES 9 C,
> three pellets three times a day.

Local treatment:
Apply CALENDULA ointment once or twice a day.

Perspiration

You shouldn't automatically try to suppress perspiration with strong anti-depressant deodorants. If the body perspires (sweats), it's because it needs to (to cool off, or because of fever, illness or stress, etc.). Suppressing perspiration artificially may induce internal disruption of the body's metabolism.
If sweating is a nuisance, it's better to reduce it with a homeopathic remedy designed to diminish sweating only insofar as is safe for the needs of the body.

Take three pellets three times a day of the remedy that best suits your needs.

Depending on the cause:
- perspiring while falling asleep,
  CALCAREA CARBONICA 9 C.
- due to obesity,
  CALCAREA CARBONICA 9 C.
- due to the slightest exercise,
  CINCHONA OFFICINALIS 9 C.
- following an acute disease,
  CINCHONA OFFICINALIS 9 C.
- from fever (sweating that doesn't bring down fever),
  MERCURIUS SOLUBILIS 9 C.
- after meals,
  NATRUM MURIATICUM 9 C.
- no apparent cause,
  PILOCARPUS 9 C.
- menopause,
  PILOCARPUS 9 C.
- on awakening,
  SAMBUCUS NIGRA 9 C.
- perspiring due to emotion,
  SEPIA 9 C.
- perspiring during menstrual periods,
  VERATRUM ALBUM 9 C.

Depending on the circumstances:
- worse at night,
  MERCURIUS SOLUBILIS 9 C.
- worse in an overheated room,
  PULSATILLA 9 C.

Depending on accompanying symptoms:
- hot sweat,
  CHAMOMILLA 9 C.
- sweats that bring on fatigue,
  CINCHONA OFFICINALIS 9 C.
- foul-smelling sweat (during spikes of fever),
  MERCURIUS SOLUBILIS 9 C.
- salty sweat (leaves white traces of salt on collars and underarms),
  NATRUM MURIATICUM 9 C.
- foul-smelling sweat under the arms,
  SEPIA 9 C.
- foul-smelling sweat on the feet,
  SILICEA 9 C.
- foul-smelling sweating of the body in general,
  THUJA OCCIDENTALIS 9 C.

▷ *Also see* **Acidity, Deodorant.**

Petroleum

Base substance: Petroleum.

Characteristic signs and symptoms:
Cracked, dirty-looking skin, particularly in winter; headaches in the occipital region; dizziness felt in the back of the head, made worse by passive movement.

Main clinical uses:
Fissuring eczema; frostbite; motion sickness; migraine headaches.

Petroselinum

Base substance: Parsley.

Characteristic signs and symptoms:
Irresistible urge to urinate; burning or itching of the urethra; milky urethral discharge.

Main clinical uses:
Chronic cystitis; urethritis; *WARNING - These diseases are serious. Contact your physician immediately for treatment recommendation.*
Urgency.

Pharyngitis (Sore throat)

Inflammation of the throat. Sore throats will benefit from the following treatments:

General treatment
- if there are bumps on the back of your sore throat, and you constantly need to clear your throat,
  ARGENTUM NITRICUM 9 C,
  three pellets three times a day.
- recurrent pharyngitis,
  BARYTA CARBONICA 9 C,
  same dosage.
- pharyngitis with yellow mucus,
  HYDRASTIS CANADENSIS 9 C,
  same dosage.

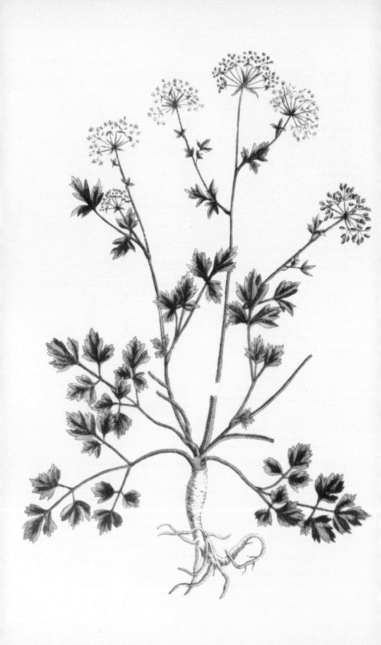

Local treatment

CALENDULA M.T.,
dissolve twenty-five drops in a glass of lukewarm pre-boiled water and gargle with this mixture twice a day.

WARNING: If your condition lasts for more than 48 hours, consult your physician.

▷ *Also see* **Rhinopharyngitis.**

A purulent sore throat may be prevented if sore throats are treated in time with:
HEPAR SULPHURIS CALCAREUM 9 C,
PYROGENIUM 9 C,
alternate three pellets of each, every two hours.
If the suppurative (pus-forming) inflammation has already reached an advanced stage, see a homeopathic physician. He or she may still be able to avoid using antibiotics. If the swelling is too great, a small incision to drain the pus may be necessary.

Philosophy

Homeopathy is based on a philosophy of respect for facts and for the laws of Nature, and respect for the priority of healing the disease before satisfying intellectual curiosity.

Phimosis

Narrowness of the foreskin of the penis preventing it from being drawn back over the glans (head of the penis). Surgical release of the tightened foreskin may be necessary. However, your doctor will be able to show you how to retract foreskin and stretch it

Petroselinum

gradually (this may avoid surgery). Phimosis is usually noticed first in young boys, and is often amenable to manual stretching.

WARNING: The condition becomes an emergency, called paraphimosis, if the retracted foreskin cannot be drawn forward again and stops blood flow to the glans. Take the child to a doctor or emergency room.

In the meantime, try:
DIOSCOREA VILLOSA 9 C,
three pellets every 15 minutes.

Phlebitis

WARNING: Check with your physician.
Inflammation of a vein, often in the legs. The leg swells and becomes painful. Bedrest and regular medical treatments are absolutely necessary. Homeopathy may profitably serve as a complementary treatment, which will be safe even with anticoagulants.

Take:
PHOSPHORUS 5 C,
PULSATILLA 5 C,
VIPERA REDII 5 C,
alternate three pellets of each, three times a day until the symptoms disappear.
"Periphlebitis" indicates inflammation of the peripheral veins, a less serious disease than the phlebitis of the deep veins. Periphlebitis may be much more responsive to the above remedies, and these may help avoid the need for anticoagulation medicines.

Phobia

▷ *See* **Neurosis, Fear.**

Phosphate in the urine

▷ *See* **Urine test.**

Phosphoricum acidum

Base substance: Phosphoric acid.
Suitable for: Mental strain.
Characteristic signs and symptoms:
Indifference due to intellectual
exhaustion; intellectual apathy;
physical exhaustion; an oppressive
sensation in the chest; light-colored
diarrhea; phosphaturia (phosphates in
the urine); loss of hair; night sweats.
Main clinical uses:
Memory loss; mental or emotional
distress; intellectual strain;
phosphaturia.

*WARNING: If condition worsens or
persists for more than 72 hours, check
with your physician.*

Phosphorus

Base substance: Phosphorus.
Suitable for:
Young people who have grown in
height rapidly and who are socially
gregarious, enthusiastic and generous.
Short periods of physical exertion tire
them easily.
Characteristic signs and symptoms:
Anxiety in the evening; a desire for
company; fear of storms; heightened
sense of smell; tendency to bleed
easily; intense hunger; intense thirst;
localized blood congestion; burning
pains; tendency to develop certain
types of lesions.
Main clinical uses:
Pulmonary congestion; laryngitis;
pancreatitis; inflammation of the
kidney; inflammations of the eye;
minor anxiety; mental or emotional
disorders; bleeding—frequent
nosebleeds, bleeding gums, heavy
menstrual periods; before surgery to
decrease the risks associated with
bleeding.

*WARNING: If condition worsens or
persists for more than 72 hours, check
with your physician.*

Phytolacca decandra

Base substance: American Nightshade,
also known as Poke.
Characteristic signs and symptoms:
Dark red throat with swollen tonsils;
burning pains in the throat radiating
to the ears; rheumatic pains from
throat inflammation; pain affecting the
inside of the thigh.
Main clinical uses:
Sore throat; pharyngitis; muscle pains;
neuralgia of the cutaneous femoris
externus nerve.

Phytotherapy

Phytotherapy is therapy using plants.
It isn't synonymous with
Homeopathy. Homeopathy not only
makes use of plants, but also animals
and minerals (see **Allopathy**).
Furthermore, the principles of
Homeopathy are not used in
phytotherapy. The Law of Similars is
not taken into account (phytotherapy
is similar to allopathy in that it aims
to combat symptoms), and
phytotherapic doses can be weighed
and measured; they are not
infinitesimal (see **Homeopathic
theory**).

Pins and needles in the extremities
(Sensation of)

Alternate three pellets of each of the following remedies, three times daily:
ACONITUM NAPELLUS 9 C,
MAGNESIA PHOSPHORICA 9 C,
PLATINUM METALLICUM 9 C.

▷ *Also see* **Hyperventilation.**

Pityriasis

Pityriasis versicolor is a common skin discoloration ailment, thought to be due to a fungus. It is usually without consequence.

Pityriasis rosea is a self-limiting (goes away on its own) outbreak of pink, raised, oval-shaped rashes that usually spare the face. This non-serious (although possibly itchy) condition can easily be diagnosed by a doctor, by virtue of a characteristic "herald patch" and a fir-tree distribution of the rashes across the back.
Take:
ARSENICUM IODATUM 9 C,
three pellets three times a day for one month.

Placebo

A placebo is a product without any therapeutic effect, which is given to patients in clinical drug trials to compare the effects of an active substance. Homeopathic physicians have performed clinical trials with placebo to check the effectiveness of homeopathic medicines and have concluded that homeopathic remedies are more active than neutral substances.

Plantago major

Base substance: the Large plantain.

Characteristic signs and symptoms:
Toothache with heavy salivation; enuresis (bed-wetting) with large amounts of urine.

Main clinical uses: Toothache; enuresis.

Platinum metallicum

Base substance: Platinum.

Suitable for:
Dark-haired, young women with a rather haughty disposition.

Characteristic signs and symptoms:
Contempt for other people; objects seem smaller than they really are; sexual arousal (mental and physical); increased sensitivity of the genital organs; constricting pains that come and go progressively; constipation when traveling.

Pleurisy (Pleuritis)

Inflammation of the pleural membrane surrounding the lungs, often with an effusion of liquid. In certain instances, this disease may respond to homeopathic treatment. Consult your doctor.

Plumbum metallicum

Base substance: Lead.

Characteristic signs and symptoms:
Violent spasmodic pain, particularly in the abdomen; constipation due to intestinal paralysis; spasms of the abdominal wall muscles which are contracted; muscular atrophy;

localized paralysis especially of the extremities, with atrophy.

Main clinical uses:
Various types of paralysis; high blood pressure; chronic kidney inflammation: *WARNING - These diseases are serious. Contact your physician immediately for treatment recommendation.*
Spasms; paralyzing sciatica; spasms of arteries in the extremities.

PMS

▷ *See* **Premenstrual syndrome.**

Pneumonia

Pneumonia is an inflammation of the lung usually from acute infection, with chest pains and occasionally coughing up of small amounts of blood. It may be amenable to homeopathic treatment by an experienced physician, but you must see a physician. Don't try to cure it on your own.

Podophyllum peltatum

Base substance: May apple or Wild mandrake.

Characteristic signs and symptoms:
Large quantities of watery diarrhea with bile; prolapse of the rectal mucosa; congestion of the liver, soothed by massaging the liver area; condition improved when lying on the stomach; symptoms worse early in the morning.

Main clinical uses:
Congestion of the liver (usually due to gallstones): *WARNING: If condition worsens or persists for more than 72 hours, check with your physician.*

Diarrhea; prolapse of the rectum; teething disorders accompanied by diarrhea.

Pollen

During pollen season many people suffer from hay fever and asthma.

▷ *See* **Asthma, Hay fever.**

Pollen

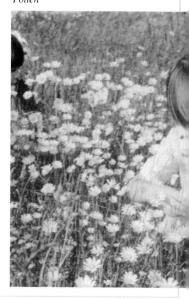

Polyps

Polyps (in the nose, uterus, bladder, colon, etc.) are not directly treatable by Homeopathy.

You must see a doctor. If the doctor believes the polyps should be removed, a complementary homeopathic treatment may also be recommended.

A long-term treatment to avoid the reappearance of polyps later should be prescribed by your homeopathic physician.

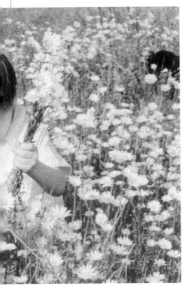

Port wine stain

▷ *See* **Angioma.**

Potentization

An essential step in the preparation of homeopathic medicines. Between each attenuation or "dilution" stage, a special laboratory instrument shakes the preparations, thereby causing molecular agitation—this is *potentization.* If omitted, the medicine will not be active.

▷ *See* **Homeopathic theory.**

Pott's disease

Tuberculosis of the spinal column (rare today). This disease must be treated by regular medicine. A homeopathic physician may prescribe a homeopathic treatment to help with some of the manifestations of the disorder, but the disease itself must be treated by some rather potent chemical medicines to achieve a cure.

Pregnancy

WARNING: As with any medication, if you are pregnant or nursing a baby, you must have professional advice.

For problems in pregnancy, take three pellets of one of the following three times a day:

For constipation during pregnancy,
COLLINSONIA CANADENSIS 9 C.

Cystitis,
POPULUS TREMULOIDES 9 C.

Diarrhea,
PHOSPHORUS 9 C.

Pain:
- for pain in the abdomen caused by the kicking of the unborn baby,
  ARNICA MONTANA 9 C.
- back pain,
  KALI CARBONICUM 9 C.
- Toothache, stomachache, pain in the breasts or head,
  SEPIA 9 C.

Fatigue, difficulty in walking,
  BELLIS PERENNIS 9 C.

False pregnancy,
  THUJA OCCIDENTALIS 9 C.

Hemorrhoids,
  COLLINSONIA CANADENSIS 9 C.

Hiccups,
  CYCLAMEN EUROPAEUM 9 C.

Irritability,
  CIMICIFUGA RACEMOSA 9 C.

Change in facial complexion,
  SEPIA 9 C.

Nausea, vomiting,
  SEPIA 9 C.

Vaginal discharge,
  SEPIA 9 C.

Fear of giving birth,
  CIMICIFUGA RACEMOSA 9 C.

Excessive saliva,
  CREOSOTUM 9 C.

Sleepiness,
  NUX MOSCHATA 9 C.

Varicose veins,
  BELLIS PERENNIS 9 C.

If any of the above treatments are not effective, look under the heading corresponding to the symptoms you are experiencing. Homeopathic medicines will not harm your unborn baby. See your doctor or gynecologist as required.

▷ *Also see* **Breast-feeding, Childbirth, Prenatal Care.**

Premature ejaculation

▷ *See* **Sexual disorders.**

Premenstrual Syndrome (PMS)

Describes the physical and/or emotional distress during the week to ten days preceding a menstrual period. This distress often virtually goes away once the flow starts and is not to be confused with other menstrual difficulties such as dysmenorrhea (extremely painful cramps); most women who experience PMS have painless, or nearly painless, periods. Symptoms of PMS are highly varied; the most common physical ones may include fatigue, weight gain, headaches, abdominal bloating and cramps, breast tenderness, food cravings, and constipation. Premenstrual tension may also lead to mood changes: from anxiety and irritability to depression.
The severity of PMS ranges from mildly troubling to almost disabling. The symptoms may change over the years and even from month to month in the same woman.

For a mild case with acute swelling and tenderness of the breasts:
  LAC CANINUM 9 C,

For a more complete symptom picture as described above:
  SEPIA 9 C.

Take three pellets three times a day, from the onset of symptoms until the first day of menstruation.

If PMS has a tendency to become chronic, lasting more than three consecutive months, discussion with a doctor may give reassurance as to the most appropriate treatment for the relief of both the physical and psychological discomfort.

Prenatal care

WARNING: As with any medication, if you are pregnant or nursing a baby, you must have professional advice. Do not take any chemical medicines during pregnancy unless you've asked your doctor.

Good prenatal care means giving your unborn baby the best treatment as possible so that he or she may be born healthy. Avoid coffee, smoking, and alcohol during pregnancy and see your doctor or gynecologist regularly. Homeopathic medicines will not harm your baby inside your body, and the following will prepare you and the baby for a healthy delivery.

Your homeopathic doctor may prescribe:

>SYPHILINUM 30 C,
MEDORRHINUM 30 C,
TUBERCULINUM NOSODE 30 C,
one unit-dose tube of each of the above every ten days in alternation (in other words, one unit-dose tube of each per month) throughout the pregnancy.

Prescriptions

Homeopathic prescriptions may vary somewhat from one doctor to the next, although for any one patient the same basic medicines should be recommended by all homeopaths. You should receive a treatment based on your individual needs, no others.

To find out what forms of homeopathic medicines to take (pellets, drops, tablets, etc.), see **Homeopathic medicines** and for prescription directions, see **When to Take the Medicine You Have Been Prescribed.**

To understand why a particular homeopathic medicine has been prescribed, you may consult *The Guide,* looking up that medicine's name (200 of the most common ones are to be found in this dictionary). By regularly referring to *The Guide,* you can better understand the why's and wherefore's of your homeopathic physician's recommendations.

Preventing diseases homeopathically

Some preventive remedies are specific to Homeopathy (see **Influenza, Mumps, Scarlatina**).

A correctly determined long-term homeopathic treatment can be an invaluable method of preventing illnesses. Your homeopathic physician will help you with this.

Prolapse

Prolapse of any of the female sexual organs can only be evaluated and treated by a gynecologist. There is no homeopathic solution.

While waiting for a gynecology consultation, take:

>ALETRIS FARINOSA 9 C,
three pellets three times a day.

Stop this treatment one week before any operation, and follow your gynecologist's instructions.

▷ *See* **Surgery.**

Prostate gland disorders

Some disorders of the prostate gland may respond to Homeopathy, particularly benign hypertrophy of the prostate gland. But you must be examined by a physician for any possible prostate problem.

Prurigo

A red, very itchy, raised rash, resembling a flea bite, that often occurs in children.
Give the child:
PULEX IRRITANS 5 C,
three pellets three times a day until symptoms disappear.

Pruritus

▷ See **Itching**.
For anal itching, ▷ see **Anus**.

Psoriasis

A scaly eruption of red, raised rashes on top of well demarcated bases, characteristically situated on the scalp, trunk, elbows, and knees. It is very difficult to treat psoriasis and a doctor should help you diagnose it.
Homeopathy is known to cure it if the treatment is started as soon as the first symptoms appear. With chronic cases, Homeopathy can only slow down the progression.
You may try taking three pellets of one of the following remedies three times a day. You should also visit a dermatologist; a medical treatment will almost certainly be needed.

Depending on how the psoriasis looks:
• desquamation (flaking off) of a fine white powder,
ARSENICUM ALBUM 9 C.
• large scales,
ARSENICUM IODATUM 9 C.
• if the skin has thickened,
GRAPHITES 9 C.
• psoriasis in round spots,
SEPIA 9 C.

Depending on the circumstances:
• itching relieved by warmth,
ARSENICUM ALBUM 9 C.

• itching aggravated by warmth,
KALI ARSENICOSUM 9 C.
• eruption of rash aggravated during winter,
PETROLEUM 9 C.
• eruption of rash aggravated during spring,
SEPIA 9 C.

Depending on the localization:
• psoriasis of the scalp,
CALCAREA CARBONICA 9 C.
• of the trunk,
KALI ARSENICOSUM 9 C.
• of the eyebrows,
PHOSPHORUS 9 C.
• of the folds of the elbow, the hollow of the knees, the face, or the nails,
SEPIA 9 C.
There is no topical homeopathic treatment for this disease. Remember to see a dermatologist.

Psorinum

Base substance: the Serous discharge of scabious vesicles.

Characteristic signs and symptoms:
Various types of itchy rashes; constant hunger, particularly the day before the onset of migraines; asthma relieved by lying down with the arms crossed over the chest; extreme cold sensitivity; lack of response to appropriate homeopathic remedies; alternating diarrhea and eczema.

Main clinical uses:
Asthma: <u>*WARNING*</u> - *This disease is serious. Contact your physician immediately for treatment recommendation.*
Tendency to catch colds; spasmodic coryza; chronic rhinitis (runny nose); migraine; eczema; the aftereffects of scabies.

Sigmund Freud (1856-1939),
the founder of psychoanalysis.

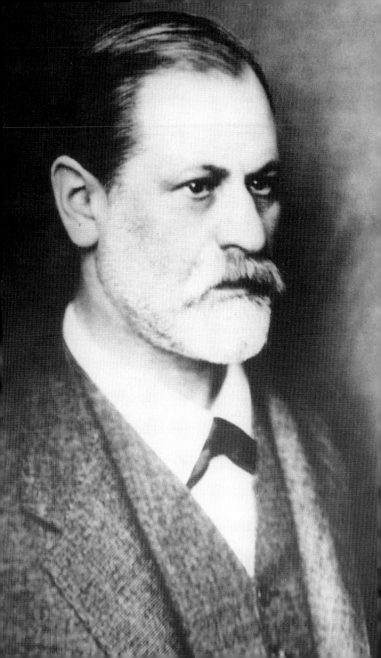

Psychiatry

Homeopathy and psychotherapy are compatible. Some types of mental diseases, however, require chemical therapy.

▷ *See* **Psychotherapy.**

Psychoanalysis

▷ *See* **Psychotherapy.**

Psychosis

Severe emotional or psychic illness, insanity. Unlike **neurosis** (see this entry), true psychosis must be treated by a psychiatrist.

▷ *Also see* **Manic depression.**

Psychosomatic disorders

Physical symptoms originating from influences of the psyche. Homeopathic treatment is effective; check with a doctor.

Psychotherapy

Psychotherapy is a therapeutic method of verbalizing problems (psychoanalysis goes even further). Psychotherapy is appropriate whenever a *need* for it is felt. In a manner of speaking, a homeopathic consultation may be a starting point for psychotherapy; Homeopathy is a field wherein symptoms of the mental sphere are held important and integrated into the general framework of all the patient's symptoms.

Homeopathic medicines that are selected with respect to a person's frame of mind are a good basis for helping psychotherapy to succeed.

Ptelea trifoliata

Base substance: Shrubby trefoil.

Characteristic signs and symptoms:
A "heavy" pain in the liver, made worse by lying on the left side; a sensation of a stone in the stomach.

Main clinical uses:
Hepatic insufficiency: *WARNING - This disease is serious. Contact your physician immediately for treatment recommendation.*
Dyspepsia.

Ptosis

▷ *See* **Eyelids.**

Puberty

If the first few menstrual periods in a pubertal woman are late or irregular, this may be normal but a physician should help to design a gentle long-term treatment that will bring about regular menstrual periods.

▷ *Also see* **Anorexia.**

If puberty is late in a boy, check with a doctor.
In the meantime, give him:
  PULSATILLA 9 C,
    three pellets three times a day.
Pubertal boys sometimes experience a feeling of *swelling* and tension in their breasts; this feeling is related to temporary hormonal reorganization. The swelling should recede on its own, without any treatment.

Pulmonary infarct

The obstruction of normal blood flow within the lung, resulting in damage to the lung tissue. Symptoms include chest pain and coughing up blood.

WARNING: This is a medical emergency; the person must have emergency medical care.

Pulsatilla

Base substance: Wind flower or Meadow anemone.

Suitable for:
Timid, emotionally prone people who blush and cry easily but who are also easily consoled; a young teen-age woman is a frequent profile.

Characteristic signs and symptoms:
Inflammation of the mucous membranes with discharge of yellow, non-irritating pus; dislike or inability to digest fats; rare thirst; generalized venous congestion; erratic pains; late menstrual periods with scant flow; morbiliform (measles-like) rash; symptoms made worse by an overheated room; a need to be outdoors; variability of symptoms.

Main clinical uses:
Styes; venous congestion; varicose veins; frostbite with changes in skin color; menstrual period disorders; puberty; various types of colds characterized by profuse, yellow nasal discharge; measles; conjunctivitis; hay fever; bronchitis; indigestion, gastric upset, flatulence, bloatedness due to eating greasy foods; rheumatism.

WARNING: If condition worsens or persists for more than 72 hours, check with your physician.

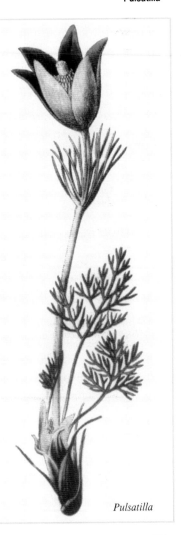

Pulsatilla

185

Pulse

An irregular pulse is not a diagnosis in itself; you should be seen by a doctor to find out its significance. Homeopathy may help to stabilize certain types of irregular pulse by integrating this symptom into the entire group of a person's symptoms.

Purpura

Hemorrhagic spots on the skin.

WARNING: They are often of serious significance and must be examined by a doctor immediately.

Pyorrhea (Parodontosis)

▷ *See* **Teeth.**

Pyrogenium

Base substance: Autolysate of animal flesh.

Characteristic signs and symptoms: Serious febrile infections with a normal pulse; bed feels hard; coated tongue.

Main clinical uses: Infections; systematic anthrax; puerperal fever: *WARNING - These diseases are serious. Contact your physician immediately for treatment recommendation.*

Qualities of a homeopathic physician

A homeopathic physician should have certain natural or acquired qualities to do his or her job best:

• humility before the facts and symptoms of human ailments (the doctor should prescribe by the symptoms he or she finds for each individual patient—not by habit or stereotyping),

• a particular sensitivity to each patient's symptoms, even the slightest ones,

• the ability to put people at ease, to have them communicate in the fullest,

• the ability to listen and to effectively integrate what people say that reflects upon their health,

• the same scientific training and background as every good doctor.

RS

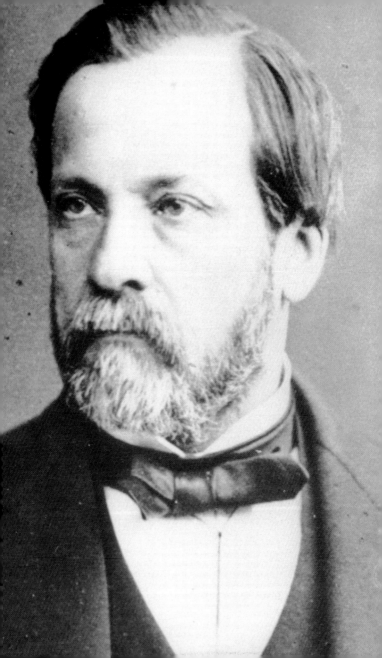

Rabies

*WARNING: Rabies is a fatal disease
unless treated early by a special
vaccine. Any animal bite should be
reported to health authorities at once.*

After the vaccine, the following
remedies may help prevent possible
side effects:
> ARSENICUM ALBUM 5 C,
> HYPERICUM PERFORATUM 5 C,
> alternate three pellets of each,
> three times a day for two months.

Ranunculus bulbosus

Base substance: the Buttercup.

Characteristic signs and symptoms:
Stabbing chest pains; bluish vesicles
on the chest wall, aggravated by
contact, exposure to cold, change in
weather and movement (particularly
breathing).

Main clinical uses:
Cutaneous herpes infections; shingles;
neuralgia after shingles; pleurisy or
pneumonia: *WARNING* - These
diseases are serious. Contact your
physician immediately for treatment
recommendation.

Raphanus sativus

Base substance: Black or garden radish.

Main clinical use:
Abdominal bloating and gas following
surgery.

Ratanhia

Base substance: Rhatany or Mapato.

Characteristic signs and symptoms:
Hemorrhoids that protrude after
passing stools; anal fissures; anal pain
persisting after passing stools; anal
spasms.

Main clinical uses:
Hemorrhoids; anal fissures; anal pain.

Raynaud's disease

*WARNING: First check with your
doctor.*
Raynaud's disease consists of arterial
spasms in the fingers of both hands,
particularly under the influence of
emotions and cold weather. The
fingers turn white, then bluish. In
most cases, the cause of this disorder
is unknown.
Before leaving home when the weather
is cold, take the following remedies:
> SECALE CORNUTUM 5 C,
> NUX VOMICA 5 C,
> AGARICUS MUSCARIUS 5 C,
> alternate three pellets of each.
> Take them as well each time you
> come in from the cold.

Reactional Mode

To the homeopathic physician,
symptoms are the expression of a
person's reactional mode. By reacting,
the body tries to ward off disease;
reactional mode is a part of vital
dynamism (see **Dynamism**).
If you swallow a poison, you vomit.
This is the body's way of reacting and
eliminating the danger. The same for
coughing if you have bronchitis; by
coughing you bring up mucus that
contains disease-causing germs. The
reactional mode signals the body's
reaction to disease.
This defense mechanism can be found
throughout nature: a pearl is no more
than an oyster's reactional symptom to

*Louis Pasteur (1822-1893),
the discoverer of the first anti-rabies vaccine, in 1886.*

a foreign body inside the shell. Mother of pearl is secreted to wall off the intruder.

▷ *See* **Symptom, Homeopathic medicines, Homeopathic theory.**

Reliability of Homeopathy

The Law of Similars is reliable; each time it is properly applied for ailments within the realm of Homeopathy, positive results are obtained.
The degree of reliability will be greater if you consult a homeopathic physician; his or her clinical experience with Homeopathy will obviously count a lot in the correct diagnosis and selection of treatments. A homeopathic doctor can individualize your case better than any book.
Homeopathic medicines themselves are highly reliable because they are prepared under careful conditions in recognized homeopathic laboratories. Doctors who are well trained both in medicine and Homeopathy exercise reliable techniques to promote and protect their patients' health (see **Homeopathic theory, Diseases, Homeopathic laboratories**).

Repertory

A repertory is an index to symptoms, listing homeopathic drug products which have produced a particular symptom in a healthy person and, if used according to the homeopathic method, will relieve a similar symptom in an ill person exhibiting this symptom. There are many repertories available, some of which may be found as computer software,

to assist homeopathic physicians in making their decisions.

▷ *See* **History of Homeopathy** (Boenninghausen, Kent).

Research
(Scientific - in Homeopathy)

For more than twenty years now, important scientific work has been and continues to be conducted in Homeopathy, as Homeopathy needs to be established on a sturdy foundation. More than a hundred research projects and scientific articles have been produced. Reports of these studies have been submitted at International Congresses and Symposia, and subsequently published in several homeopathic journals.
This research demonstrates the biological and pharmaceutical activity of Hahnemannian potencies and their curative and preventive action against diseases experimentally induced in laboratory plants and animals.

Retention of Urine

▷ *See* **Urinating.**

Rheum

Base substance: Rhubarb.

Characteristic signs and symptoms: Acidic diarrhea; cold sweats with an acidic odor.

Main clinical uses: Diarrhea; teething disorders.

Rheumatism (Joint Pains)

Acute articular rheumatism is sometimes due to a strep throat.

Anytime your children (or you) have a red, sore throat you should show it to a physician. (He or she should perform a throat culture.)

Rheumatism may be treatable by Homeopathy, but is approaching its limits. You must speak to a doctor who is knowledgeable of rheumatic diseases (family doctor, internist, rheumatologist) as well as of Homeopathy. Follow his or her advice even if they recommend antibiotics or other medicines. The complications of acute rheumatic fever can be long-term and serious if not prevented.

Inflammatory rheumatism (arthritis):

This is an auto-immune disease. Consult your doctor or rheumatologist.

▷ *See* **Rheumatoid arthritis.**

Joint pains:

For joint pains, take three pellets of one or more of the following remedies three times a day.

Depending on the cause:
- joint pains caused by getting wet,
  DULCAMARA 9 C.
- after a chill,
  NUX VOMICA 9 C.
- after physical strain,
  RHUS TOXICODENDRON 9 C.

Depending on the modifying circumstances:
Improvement:
- when it rains,
  CAUSTICUM 9 C.
- when the weather is cold,
  LEDUM PALUSTRE 9 C.
- by warmth or heat,
  RHUS TOXICODENDRON 9 C.
- by moving around, walking or "loosening up,"
  RHUS TOXICODENDRON 9 C.

Aggravation:
- during menstrual periods,
  CIMICIFUGA RACEMOSA 9 C.
- by walking, moving around,
  BRYONIA ALBA 9 C.

- when it snows,
  CALCAREA PHOSPHORICA 9 C.
- when it rains or when the weather is wet,
  DULCAMARA 9 C.
- at night,
  KALI IODATUM 9 C.
- by change of weather or when there's a storm,
  RHODODENDRON CHRYSANTHEMUM 9 C.
- when resting,
  RHUS TOXICODENDRON 9 C.

Depending on the accompanying symptoms:
- alternating rheumatism and diarrhea,
  ARTEMISIA ABROTANUM 9 C.
- muscle pains and other pains not related to the bones,
  CIMICIFUGA RACEMOSA 9 C.
- joint pain with painless swelling,
  APIS MELLIFICA 9 C.
- joint pain with painful swelling,
  BRYONIA ALBA 9 C.
- with stiffness,
  CAUSTICUM ANNUUM 9 C.
- alternating joint pains and gastritis,
  KALI BICHROMICUM 9 C.
- unpredictable onset of joint pains,
  KALI SULPHURICUM 9 C.
- joint pain with cramps,
  NUX VOMICA 9 C.
- with numbness,
  RHUS TOXICODENDRON 9 C.
- pain in the tendons,
  RHUS TOXICODENDRON 9 C.

Depending on the localization of joint pains:
see the heading corresponding to the part of the body.

Gout:
▷ *see* this entry.

Rheumatoid arthritis

Rheumatoid arthritis should be diagnosed and treated by a medical doctor or rheumatologist.

The early stages of this disease, however, may benefit from a homeopathic treatment. Your homeopathic doctor may advise you to take:

STREPTOCOCCIN NOSODE 12 C, three unit-dose tubes a week for several months, even years.

Rhinopharyngitis
(Runny nose and sore throat)

Children suffering from inflammation of the nose and the back of the throat should be given three pellets of one or more of the following remedies throughout the acute period.

Depending on the type of nasal and throat secretion:
- yellow secretion, which irritates the upper lip,
  ARSENICUM IODATUM 9 C.
- foul-smelling secretion,
  HEPAR SULPHURIS CALCAREUM 9 C.
- chunks of yellow phlegm, particularly at the back of the throat,
  HYDRASTIS CANADENSIS 9 C.
- greenish-yellow, stringy secretion,
  KALI BICHROMICUM 9 C.
- scabs inside the nose,
  KALI BICHROMICUM 9 C.
- grayish-white secretion,
  KALI MURIATICUM 9 C.
- yellow, chronic secretion,
  KALI SULPHURICUM.
- irritating, greenish-yellow secretion,
  MERCURIUS SOLUBILIS 9 C.
- watery, almost yellow, non-irritating secretion,
  PULSATILLA 9 C.

Stopped up nose (nasal congestion):
- nose stopped up and runny at the same time,
  NUX VOMICA 9 C.
- nasal congestion at night,
  NUX VOMICA 9 C.
- nasal congestion in an overheated room,
  PULSATILLA 9 C.

- nose is stopped up and dry,
  SAMBUCUS NIGRA 9 C.
- for children who sniff constantly,
  SAMBUCUS NIGRA 9 C.

Rhinopharyngitis with otitis (ear infection): (WARNING - You must check with your physician.)
AGRAPHIS NUTANS 5 C.
Ear infections often recur in young children. Check with a homeopathic physician; he or she will be able to prescribe a long-term treatment.

Rhododendron chrysanthemum

Base substance: the Rhododendron.

Characteristic signs and symptoms: Rheumatism; toothache; testicular pain; aggravation of symptoms during stormy weather.

Main clinical uses:
Inflammation of the testicles:
WARNING - This disease is serious. You should consult your physician for advice.
Gout; joint pains; headache.

Rhus aromatica

Base substance: Fragrant sumac.

Main clinical use:
Enuresis (bed-wetting) due to atony (lack of muscle tone) of the bladder.

Rhus toxicodendron

Base substance: Poison ivy or Poison sumac.

Suitable for: Consequences of overexertion.

Characteristic signs and symptoms:
Joint stiffness; swollen painful joints,
aggravated by start of motions and
improved by continuing movement;
joint pains aggravated by exposure to
wet cold; itchy, fluid-filled (vesicular)
rashes; inflammation of the mucous
membranes; dreams of tiring exercise.

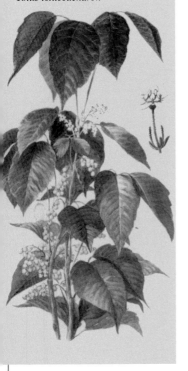

Rhus toxicodendron

Main clinical uses:
Flu-like symptoms with fever,
diarrhea, generalized body pains and
stiffness, and thirst for cold water or
milk; colds; laryngitis; sprain;
tendinitis; joint pain; excess muscle
fatigue; lumbago; sciatica; hives;
eczema; chicken pox.

*WARNING: If condition worsens or
persists for more than 72 hours, check
with your physician.*

Ricinus communis

Base substance: the Castor-oil plant.
Characteristic signs and symptoms:
Feeling as if a metal rod were across
the stomach; painless diarrhea;
excessive lactation of the breasts, or
lack of breast-milk.
Main clinical uses:
Gastroenteritis; stimulation of
maternal lactation.

Rickets

*WARNING: You must check with your
doctor.*
Rickets is a calcium-deficiency disease
occurring in children. Some of the
main symptoms are: late closing of the
fontanelles, enlarging of the wrists, a
hollow in the sternum, saddle knees, a
"rosary" of bony bumps on the rib
cage.
Make sure your child has proper
nourishment and have the child
checked by a homeopathic physician.
If you have doubts or if you suspect
rickets, you may give:
CALCAREA PHOSPHORICA 6 X,
SILICEA 6 X,
two tablets of each, three times a
day.

193

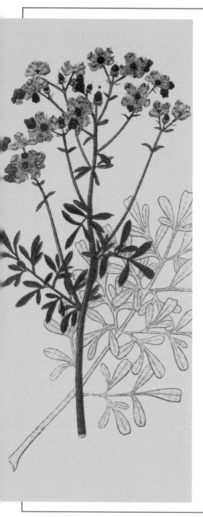

Ringing in the ears

WARNING: If the ringing won't go away (or if you feel dizzy or lose your balance), you must check with your doctor. You might be suffering from an acute ear disorder that needs immediate treatment.

For ringing or humming in the ears, take:

> CHININUM SULPHURICUM 9 C,
> NATRUM SALICYLICUM 9 C,
> alternate three pellets of each, three times a day.

Robinia

Base substance: the Yellow locust or False acacia plant.

Main clinical use:
Stomachburn with acidic vomiting.

Rosacea (Acne)

▷ *See* **Acne.**

Rumex crispus

Base substance: Yellow dock.

Main clinical use:
Coughing from breathing in cold air, even minute amounts.

Ruta graveolens

Base substance: the Rue or Bitter herb.

Characteristic signs and symptoms:
Bruising pain all over; bone and tendon pain with contractures, particularly in the thighs and wrists; eye muscle fatigue; rectal prolapse.

Main clinical uses:
Traumatism to a ligament; stiffness and contusion in the limbs and joints; tendinitis; wrist pain; lumbago; sciatica; muscle strain and sprains; visual fatigue, eye strain.

WARNING: If condition worsens or persists for more than 72 hours, check with your physician.

Sabadilla

Base substance: Cevadilla seeds.

Characteristic signs and symptoms:
Violent sneezing; sensitivity (aversion) to the smell of flowers; sensation of a lump in the throat with a constant urge to swallow; anal itching.

Main clinical uses:
Hay fever; spasmodic coryza. Intestinal worms (such as pinworms): *WARNING - This disease is serious. Contact your physician immediately for treatment recommendation.*

Sabal serrulata

Base substance: the fruit of Saw palmetto, a North American palm tree.

Characteristic signs and symptoms:
Enlarged prostate gland with urinary difficulty and painful sexual intercourse.

Main clinical uses:
Prostate disorders; sexual disorders: *WARNING - These diseases are serious. Contact your physician immediately for treatment recommendation.*
Cystitis.

Sabina

Base substance: the Savin juniper.

Characteristic signs and symptoms:
Migrating pains from the sacrum to the pubis; anterior thigh pain when walking; heavy menstrual periods; uterine bleeding.

Main clinical uses:
Menstrual period pains; risk of miscarriage in the third month of pregnancy; leg or thigh neuralgia.

Saliva

Too much:
MERCURIUS SOLUBILIS 9 C,
three pellets three times a day.

Absence of, or too little:
NUX MOSCHATA 9 C,
same dosage.

Thick, cottony:
BERBERIS VULGARIS 9 C,
same dosage.

Salivary glands

Abscess:
MERCURIUS SOLUBILIS 9 C,
PYROGENIUM 9 C,
alternate three pellets of each,
three times a day.

Ranula (sublingual cyst, destruction of
a salivary gland beneath the tongue):
AMBRA GRISEA 9 C,
THUJA OCCIDENTALIS 9 C,
alternate three pellets of each,
three times a day.

Sambucus nigra

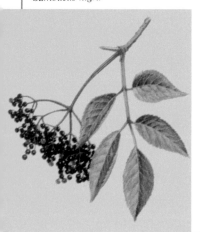

Salpingitis

*WARNING: Check with your
physician before any treatment. The
diagnosis of inflammation of the
fallopian tubes must be made by a
doctor.*

While waiting for your doctor's advice,
take the following:
MERCURIUS SOLUBILIS 9 C,
three pellets three times a day, and
get as much rest as you can.

Sambucus nigra

Base substance: Black elder.

Characteristic signs and symptoms:
Child who wakes suddenly at night
with congestion, stridor, cough, and a
great deal of perspiration.

Main clinical uses:
Laryngeal stridor or false croup;
coryza.

*WARNING: If condition worsens or
persists for more than 72 hours, check
with your physician.*

Sanguinaria canadensis

Base substance: Blood root.

Characteristic signs and symptoms:
Localized vascular congestion (head,
cheeks, hands, feet); throbbing
headache with red cheeks, hot flashes,
relieved by passing gas or burping;
burning mucous membranes; bleeding
polyps; dry cough relieved by burping.

Main clinical indications:
Migraines; facial neuralgia;
palpitations; hot flashes; menopause;
polyps; coryza.

Sarsaparilla

Base substance: Sarsaparilla.

Characteristic signs and symptoms:
Violent pains at the end of
micturation; urine comes out drop by
drop; urinating is easier while standing
up; white urates in the urine; dry,
cracked, flaccid skin; aggravation of
symptoms by humidity and in the
spring.

Main clinical uses:
Urinary stones; renal colic (kidney
stones): *WARNING - These diseases
are serious. Contact your physician
immediately for treatment
recommendation.*
Chronic cystitis.

Scabies

To cure this parasitic disease you will
first need a regular medical treatment.
See your doctor, and also take:
PSORINUM 30 C,
one weekly unit-dose tube, over a
period of three months. This will
help to avoid relapses.

Scalp

Crusts on child's scalp (cradle cap):
CALCAREA CARBONICA 9 C,
three pellets three times a day,
without fail.
- If the scalp smells bad:
  HEPAR SULPHURIS CALCAREUM 9 C,
  alternate three pellets of this, three
  times a day, with the above.
- If the scalp itches:
  MEZEREUM 9 C,
  alternate three pellets of this, three
  times a day, with the above.
- When the scalp itches for no
  apparent reason:
  OLEANDER 9 C,
  three pellets three times a day.

- If the scalp is painful:
  OLEANDER 9 C,
  three pellets three times a day.

Eczema:
GRAPHITES 9 C,
VIOLA TRICOLOR 9 C,
alternate three pellets of each,
three times a day, until your
homeopathic physician can
prescribe a long-term preventive
treatment.

Sebaceous cyst:
BARYTA CARBONICA 9 C,
three pellets three times a day.
This treatment will *prevent* sebaceous
cysts from forming but won't get rid of
existing ones; have them removed
only if they are unsightly or
bothersome.

Psoriasis: ▷ *see* this entry.

Greasy seborrhea:
OLEANDER 9 C,
three pellets three times a day.

Scarlatina (Scarlet Fever)

For scarlatina, an acute disease with
fever and red rash (frequent in
children), a physician must carefully
choose the remedy indicated by the
symptoms. If not, there is a risk of
complications.

*WARNING: See a doctor without fail
(even if you take a homeopathic
medicine). If the homeopathic
physician wants you to take antibiotics,
take them.*

Preventing scarlatina:
When one member of the family is
suffering from scarlatina, give any
children who are in contact with the
patient:
STREPTOCOCCIN NOSODE 9 C,
three pellets, three times a day for
two weeks.

Scars

To make scars less visible, to help
them heal, or to treat possible
complications, take three pellets three
times a day of one of the following
medicines.

Knobby scars,
   GRAPHITES 9 C.
GRAPHITES ointment is also
recommended, but it is dark and may
stain. You may prefer to use it at night
as a dressing.

Keloids (raised scars),
   GRAPHITES 9 C.

Scars resulting from burns,
   CAUSTICUM 9 C.

Color:
- if the scars are red,
   LACHESIS 9 C.
- if the scars are blue,
   SULPHURICUM ACIDUM 9 C.

Itching around the scar,
   FLUORICUM ACIDUM 9 C.

Scars that hurt:
- because of dry weather,
   CAUSTICUM 9 C.
- along the nerves,
   HYPERICUM PERFORATUM 9 C.
- because of a change in weather,
   NITRICUM ACIDUM 9 C.
- because of damp weather,
   PHYTOLACCA DECANDRA 9 C.

Scars surrounded by blisters,
   FLUORICUM ACIDUM 9 C.

To help scar healing after an operation,
   STAPHYSAGRIA 9 C.
   (The treatment should last until
   the scar is completely healed.)

Scars that open up and ooze,
   SILICEA 9 C.

Scars that bleed,
   LACHESIS 9 C.

Scheuermann's disease
(Growth epiphysitis)

WARNING: Check with your doctor.

This is a benign, adolescent growth
disorder of the vertebrae. It is
sometimes painful.
Treat pain by consulting the heading,
Rheumatism and systematically
supplement the remedy you have
chosen with the following:
   CALCAREA PHOSPHORICA 6 X,
   two tablets, three times a day as
   long as pain lasts.

Schizophrenia

A psychosis characterized by loss of
contact with reality. This disease may
be responsive to Homeopathy but only
in its early stages. If possible, consult a
homeopathic psychiatrist.

Schuessler's salts

▷ *See* **Cell salts (Schuessler's).**

Sciatica

Nerve pain running from the lumbar
region to the foot via the back of the
thigh, or the leg.
Only rheumatic sciatica may be
treated homeopathically. If sciatica is
due to a herniated disk, it may have to
be dealt with surgically. Take three
pellets of one or more of the following
remedies three times daily.

Depending on circumstances:
Aggravated:
- when sitting,
   AMMONIUM MURIATICUM 9 C.

- on the slightest movement,
  BRYONIA ALBA 9 C.
- at night,
  KALI IODATUM 9 C.
- when resting, in bed,
  RHUS TOXICODENDRON 9 C.
- by exposure to humidity,
  RHUS TOXICODENDRON 9 C.
- when standing,
  SULPHUR 9 C.
- by coughing, sneezing or when
  passing stools,
  TELLURIUM 9 C.

Improved:
- by lying on the painful side,
  BRYONIA ALBA 9 C.
- by bending the leg upward,
  COLOCYNTHIS 9 C.
- by sitting,
  GNAPHALIUM POLYCEPHALUM 9 C.
- by pressing on the leg,
  MAGNESIA PHOSPHORICA 9 C.
- by heat,
  MAGNESIA PHOSPHORICA 9 C.
- by moving around or walking,
  RHUS TOXICODENDRON 9 C.

Depending on sensations:
- a burning sensation which is relieved
  by heat,
  ARSENICUM ALBUM 9 C.
- prickly pains,
  BRYONIA ALBA 9 C.
- numbness,
  GNAPHALIUM POLYCEPHALUM 9 C.
- pain seems to move along the leg,
  KALI BICHROMICUM 9 C.
- a sensation of an electric current,
  KALMIA LATIFOLIA 9 C.
- sciatica moving from one side to the
  other and back again,
  LAC CANINUM 9 C.
- shooting pains,
  MAGNESIA PHOSPHORICA 9 C.
- a sensation of cramps,
  NUX VOMICA 9 C.

Depending on accompanying symptoms:
- paralyzing sciatica,
  CAUSTICUM ANNUUM 9 C.
- sciatica with muscular atrophy,
  PLUMBUM METALLICUM 9 C.

Scientific research in Homeopathy

▷ *See* **Research (Scientific - in Homeopathy).**

Scilla maritima

Base substance: the Squill or Sea
Onion.
Characteristic signs and symptoms:
Coughing with sneezing; watering of
the eyes; involuntary passing of urine
and stools; sharp pains in the chest.
Main clinical uses:
Whooping cough: *WARNING - This
disease is serious. You must consult
your physician for treatment
recommendation.*
Coryza; bronchial colds.

Sclerosing injections of varicose veins and hemorrhoids

Sclerosing injections designed to
harden and obturate veins are both
illogical and ill-advised. Illogical,
because they don't solve the
underlying problems of venous
circulation; the sclerosed vein may
disappear but a nearby vein might
swell up. Ill-advised, because once all
the troublesome veins have been
sclerosed, secondary infections or skin
problems might set in.
The symptoms of hemorrhoids and
varicose veins may be effectively
treated by Homeopathy. As for
aesthetics, they should sometimes take
second place to the respect of natural
principles. Discuss your case with your
physician.

Scoliosis

For pains resulting from scoliosis, see
Spinal column.
The correction of scoliosis does not lie
within the field of Homeopathy.

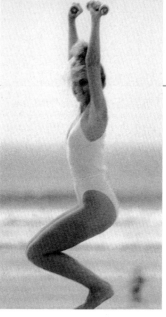

*Keep your spinal column in good
shape with regular exercise.*

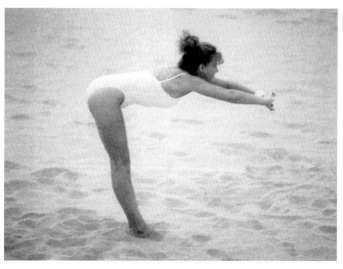

Sea climate (Intolerance to)

If you feel nervous, exhausted, drowsy or suffer from insomnia when staying near the sea, the best solution is to not go there in the first place! If you must spend some time at the seaside, try not to stay more than a week or ten days. While you are there, take:
NATRUM MURIATICUM 9 C,
three pellets three times a day.

For seasickness, ▷ *see* **Travel sickness.**

Sebaceous cysts

▷ See **Scalp.**

Seborrhea

▷ See **Scalp.**

Secale cornutum

Base substance: Spurred rye (or ergot).
Characteristic signs and symptoms: Burning pains; skin is cold to the touch but pain is made worse by exposure to heat; a sensation of "pins and needles"; tendency to gangrene; serious infection; green diarrhea.

Main clinical uses:
Arterial spasms; early stages of gangrene; Raynaud's disease:
WARNING - These diseases are serious. You must consult your physician for treatment recommendation.
Diarrhea.

Selenium

Base substance: Selenium.
Main clinical uses: Acne with blackheads.

Self-medication

Is there any danger in treating yourself by Homeopathy?

In other words, can you use *The Guide* to treat your health problems without risk? The main risk is obviously to look at the wrong heading, and falsely diagnose an illness. With careful reading, this will not happen. In many cases, the disease will merely be a relapse of a former one and the doctor will have already told you its name. Of course, in case of a serious condition, consult your doctor immediately.
Even if you should make a mistake and choose the wrong homeopathic medicine, there is no danger.
Homeopathic medicines are not toxic, as some medicines can be. This doesn't mean that homeopathic remedies are **placebos** (that is, harmless inert substances given as if they were medicines). They are active medicines, but only when they correspond exactly to the symptoms of your ailment. You might liken this to a lock that can only be opened with the right key.
You should always consult your doctor if you have any doubts about a health problem. The advice given in *The Guide* is not an excuse to bypass the clinical judgement of your doctor.

Are there any advantages to self-medication?

Self-medication will enable you to best get through the period preceding your doctor's appointment. If you obtain good results with one of the treatment recommendations in *The Guide,* you may still wish to have the benefit of your homeopathic doctor's experience. This can be a basis for wider understanding of good health decisions.

Senecio aureus

Base substance: Golden Senecio, or Liferoot.

Main clinical use:
Heavy menstrual periods with compensation phenomena (nosebleeds, white vaginal discharge, colds, lumbago).

Senile coxarthritis
(Hip arthritis)

▷ *See* **Hips.**

Senna

Base substance: Cassia, or Senna.

Main clinical use:
Ketoacidosis: *WARNING - This disease is serious. You must contact your physician immediately for treatment recommendation. (Always necessitates emergency medical care).*

Sepia

Base substance: Squid ink (Cuttlefish).

Suitable for:
Postpartum women with rings under their eyes, who are exhausted and depressed from multiple pregnancies.

Characteristic signs and symptoms:
Irritability which is aggravated by being consoled; an aversion to company, work; problems coping with family; lack of sexual desire; tiredness for no special reason; hot flashes (even before menopause); herpes during menstrual periods; cold sensitivity, aggravated by being near the sea and when it snows; an empty feeling in the pit of the stomach around 11 a.m.; a craving for sugar, chocolate, lemons and vinegar; a sensation of heaviness in the pelvis; strong-smelling urine; round rashes that heal from the center outward.

Main clinical uses:
Frigidity; impotency; urinary infection; herpes; jaundice; hepatic insufficiency: *WARNING - These diseases are serious. Contact your physician immediately for treatment recommendation.*
Mental or emotional strain; cystitis; menstrual or premenstrual disorders; disorders due to pregnancy and childbirth; constipation; hemorrhoids; migraines; spasmophilia; acne rosacea.

Septicemia

Certain forms of septicemia (bacterial infection of the bloodstream) may respond to a homeopathic treatment. Consult your homeopathic physician.

WARNING: Septicemia is a potentially life-threatening illness that must always be treated as an emergency by a medical doctor.

Sexual disorders

Take three pellets of the remedy you have chosen twenty days per month. Check with a homeopathic physician if self-medication doesn't seem to be working.

An aversion to sexual intercourse:
  GRAPHITES 9 C.

Continence (disorders related to chastity, virginity, celibacy):
  CONIUM MACULATUM 9 C.

Desire:
• if it's lacking,
  ONOSMODIUM VIRGINIANUM 9 C.
• if it's excessive,
  PLATINUM METALLICUM 9 C.

Pain during intercourse:
- in case of cramps occurring before ejaculation,
  CAUSTICUM ANNUUM 9 C.
- in case of vaginal pain from dryness,
  LYCOPODIUM CLAVATUM 9 C.

Premature ejaculation:
  SELENIUM 9 C.

Erection (difficulty in obtaining an):
- erection is lost as soon as penetration is attempted,
  ARGENTUM NITRICUM 9 C.
- erection is impossible despite desire,
  CALADIUM SEGUINUM 9 C.
- painful erection while sleeping,
  CANTHARIS 9 C.
- erection is impossible despite erotic thoughts,
  SELENIUM 9 C.

Sexual arousal, constant sexual ideas:
  STAPHYSAGRIA 9 C.

Sexual excesses:
  SELENIUM 9 C,
  for all disorders which may result from the above.

Exhibitionism: consult both a psychiatrist and a homeopathic physician.

Fatigue after sexual intercourse:
  LYCOPODIUM CLAVATUM 9 C.

Frigidity: ▷ *see* the paragraphs "Desire" and "Pleasure."

Impotence: ▷ *see* the paragraphs "Desire," "Ejaculation," "Erection," and "Pleasure."

Masturbation: there is no treatment. It is not an illness.

Nymphomania: ▷ *see* the paragraph "Desire."

Fear of having sexual intercourse, fear of members of the opposite sex:
  PULSATILLA 9 C.

Pleasure:
- lack of,
  CALADIUM SEGUINUM 9 C.
- delayed,
  KALI PHOSPHORICUM 9 C.

Wet dreams:
- spontaneous ejaculation due to sexual ideas,
  CONIUM MACULATUM 9 C.
- spontaneous wet dreams,
  PICRICUM ACIDUM 9 C.

Vaginismus: ▷ *see* this entry. Speak with your homeopathic physician; sexual symptoms are a part of medicine.

▷ *Also see* **Psychotherapy.**

Shingles (Herpes zoster)

WARNING: Check with your doctor.
The homeopathic treatment for shingles may be very effective provided it is started as soon as the rash erupts. Shingles causes a series of small, painful vesicles along a nerve path, most often on the trunk. Once the painful stage is reached, the treatment result is only partial.

When the rash has just started to break, take:
  ARSENICUM ALBUM 30 C,
  one unit-dose tube as soon as possible (do not repeat);
then,
  MEZEREUM 9 C,
  RANUNCULUS BULBOSUS 9 C,
  RHUS TOXICODENDRON 9 C,
  alternate three pellets of each, three times a day over a period of three weeks.

If the painful stage has been reached (you might avoid this stage with earlier homeopathic treatment), take three pellets of one of the following remedies three times a day:
- for a burning sensation in the area of the shingles (relieved by heat),
  ARSENICUM ALBUM 9 C.
- shooting pains along the affected nerve,
  KALMIA LATIFOLIA 9 C.

- strong pain,
    MEZEREUM 9 C.
- a burning sensation made worse by heat,
    MEZEREUM 9 C.
- pain aggravated by touching, bathing, or at night,
    MEZEREUM 9 C.

Shivering

Does the person also have a fever? Take his or her temperature. Fever with shivering should be reported to a doctor. Note the times that the shivering episodes occur. This will make it much easier for your doctor to decide on the suitable remedy.

Shock

Emotional, sentimental, mental: ▷ *see* **Emotion.**

Post-operative shock: ▷ *see* **Surgery.**

▷ *Also see* **Trauma.**

Shortness of breath
(Dyspnea)

Difficulty or distress in breathing (frequently rapid breathing) may or may not be associated with diseases of the heart or lungs.

WARNING: It is important that you see your doctor.

Take three pellets of one or more of the following remedies three times a day for:
- shortness of breath from exertion,
    ARNICA MONTANA 9 C.
- shortness of breath when you swallow,
    BROMIUM 9 C.
- shortness of breath because of digestion-related bloating,
    CARBO VEGETABILIS 9 C.

- shortness of breath when coughing,
    DROSERA ROTUNDIFOLIA 9 C.
- shortness of breath when falling asleep,
    GRINDELIA ROBUSTA 9 C.
- shortness of breath when anxious or nervous,
    IGNATIA AMARA 9 C.
- shortness of breath when a handkerchief is about to cover your nose, or when your hand or scarf touchs your neck,
    LACHESIS 9 C.
- shortness of breath during wet weather,
    NATRUM SULPHURICUM 9 C.
- shortness of breath during menstrual periods,
    SPONGIA TOSTA 9 C.

▷ For shortness of breath due to **asthma** or **bronchitis,** *see* these entries.

Shoulder

For pains in the shoulder, look under the heading, **Rheumatism,** and add:
    FERRUM METALLICUM 9 C,
    three pellets three times a day.

Silicea

Base substance: Silica.

Suitable for:
Children with growth problems, trouble assimilating knowledge, and problems with demineralization; the aftereffects of vaccinations.

Characteristic signs and symptoms:
Lack of mental and physical energy; lack of self-confidence; suppuration of the smallest wounds; foul-smelling sweating of the feet; constipation with stools that partially leave the rectum and return; cold sensitivity.

Main clinical uses:
Suppuration; sinusitis; chronic bronchitis; pyorrhea; fistula.

<u>WARNING</u>: *If condition worsens or persists for more than 72 hours, check with your physician.*

Similars (Law of)

The Law of Similars is the experimental basis of Homeopathy : certain substances are capable of curing illnesses similar to those they themselves produce.

▷ *See* **Homeopathic theory.**

Simillimum

This means the best medicine adapted to the case in question. The *simillimum* is determined by applying the Law of Similars (see **Homeopathic theory**). *Simillimum* is Latin for "the most similar." This brings us back to the idea that although several remedies may seem suitable for a particular case, one of them will fit the symptoms better than the others. This one is the *simillimum.*

Sinusitis

Inflammation of the sinuses.

For acute sinusitis, take three pellets of one or more of the following remedies three times a day:
● sinusitis without nasal secretions but with stopped-up nose,
    BELLADONNA 9 C.
● painful sinusitis that is made worse by touching,
    HEPAR SULPHURIS CALCAREUM 9 C.
● aggravated by the slightest draft of air,
    HEPAR SULPHURIS CALCAREUM 9 C.

● with thick, yellow, stringy nasal secretions that are almost rubbery,
    HYDRASTIS CANADENSIS 9 C.
● with green secretion or crusts in the nose,
    KALI BICHROMICUM 9 C.
● with pus mixed with blood from the nose, (See your doctor.)
    PHOSPHORUS 9 C.

For chronic sinusitis, try:
    SILICEA 9 C,
    three pellets three times a day.
Should the above treatments fail to give positive results, consult a homeopathic doctor. A long-term treatment may be more effective in preventing sinusitis.

Skin

The treatment of skin diseases is one field in which Homeopathy is highly successful.

▷ *Look under* the following headings: **Abscess, Acne, Anthrax, Eczema, Erysipelas, Frostbite, Herpes, Impetigo, Injuries, Itching, Mycosis, Perspiration, Psoriasis, Scars, Shingles, Sun, Urticaria, Warts, Whitlow.**

▷ For the local use of ointments, *see* **Ointments.**

Sleep (Symptoms during)

Take three pellets of the selected remedy three times a day.
Singing:
    CROCUS SATIVUS 9 C.

Shouting:
    APIS MELLIFICA 9 C.

Enuresis:
▷ *see* this entry.
Grinding of the teeth:
    BELLADONNA 9 C.

Chewing:
    BRYONIA ALBA 9 C.

Stopped-up nose:
    SAMBUCUS NIGRA 9 C.

Talking:
    BELLADONNA 9 C.

Crying:
    CHAMOMILLA 9 C.

Pruritus, anal itching:
    COFFEA CRUDA 9 C.

Laughing:
    LYCOPODIUM CLAVATUM 9 C.

Sleepwalking:
▷ *see* this entry.

Sensation of suffocation:
• when falling asleep,
    GRINDELIA ROBUSTA 9 C.
• while asleep,
    LACHESIS 9 C.

Waking up suddenly (startled):
• when falling asleep,
    BELLADONNA 9 C.
• while asleep,
    HYOSCYAMUS NIGER 9 C.

Nightmares:
    STRAMONIUM 9 C.

Sweating:
    CHAMOMILLA 9 C.

Eyes half-open:
    LYCOPODIUM CLAVATUM 9 C.

▷ *Also see* **Insomnia, Drowsiness.**

Sleepwalking

This nervous disorder is not as serious as some parents think. Also, it won't hurt your child to be awaken and led back to bed.

As a preventive treatment, try:
    KALI BROMATUM 9 C,
    STRAMONIUM 9 C,
    alternate three pellets of each, three times a day, twenty days a month over a period of three months.

Slow action

Does Homeopathy, as it's often said, work slowly?
With recent acute cases, Homeopathy works very rapidly. In the case of chronic diseases, homeopathic treatment *seems* to act slowly for there are rarely immediate results. On the other hand, Homeopathy makes it possible to cure diseases in just a few years, which would otherwise have lasted throughout the patient's entire life.

Slow-wittedness: ▷ *see* **Lymphatism.**

Smell (Sense of)

▷ *See* **Nose.**

Snake bites

<u>*WARNING:*</u> *If you or a child are bitten by a snake, you must immediately head for a hospital or doctor.*

If it's impossible to determine whether the snake was poisonous, you should still seek medical care and follow these instructions on the way:
- try to keep the patient calm and immobilize the bitten part of the body. Use a tourniquet to slow down blood and lymph flow but remember to loosen it every now and then.
- suck on the bite, if you see it, to remove venom (with a suction bulb for this purpose if you have one, or with your mouth if you have no open cuts on your lips or in your mouth). If the area around the bite has started to swell rapidly, you may have to make a small skin incision above the swollen

area and suck, if you are familiar with this technique (and if you're far from a doctor's help).
- above all, keep the patient calm and still and get to a doctor or hospital.

Sneezing

▷ *See* **Colds.**

Snow-blindness

Snow-blindness (irritation of the eye caused by ultraviolet sunrays reflected by the snow):
ACONITUM NAPELLUS 9 C,
APIS MELLIFICA 9 C,
alternate three pellets of each, three times a day.

Beware of cheap and ineffective sunglasses available in non-specialized stores. They often protect your eyes only from the glare of the sun, and not from the ultraviolet rays.

Solidago virgaurea

Base substance: Golden rod.

Characteristic signs and symptoms: Kidney pain; small quantities of clear, foul-smelling urine.

Main clinical uses:
Kidney stones: *WARNING - This disease is serious. Contact your physician immediately for treatment recommendation.*
Difficulty in urinating.

Sore Throat, Tonsillitis

WARNING: If this condition persists more than 24 to 48 hours, see your physician.

The homeopathic treatment for a severe inflammatory or ulcerated condition of the throat is as follows:

Depending on the symptoms:
- for a bright red sore throat,
  BELLADONNA 9 C,
  MERCURIUS SOLUBILIS 9 C,
  alternate three pellets of each, three times a day.
- for a dark red sore throat,
  PHYTOLACCA DECANDRA 9 C,
  three pellets three times a day.
- for a sore throat with pain radiating to the ears or the nape of the neck,
  PHYTOLACCA DECANDRA 9 C,
  three pellets three times a day.
- for a sore throat covered with white spots,
  MERCURIUS SOLUBILIS 9 C,
  three pellets three times a day.
- when only the left tonsil is affected,
  LACHESIS 9 C,
  three pellets three times a day, to supplement one of the above treatments.
- when only the right tonsil is affected,
  LYCOPODIUM CLAVATUM 9 C,
  three pellets three times a day, to supplement one of the above treatments.
- if a tonsillar inflammation with pus seems likely, (Check with your doctor.)
  HEPAR SULPHURIS CALCAREUM 9 C,
  three pellets three times a day, to supplement one of the above treatments.

Gargle two or three times a day with: twenty-five drops of CALENDULA M.T. in a glass of pre-boiled lukewarm water.

Is the homeopathic treatment for acute sore throat dangerous?

An incorrectly treated sore throat can lead to other complications (kidney infections or nephritis, acute rheumatic fever of the joints). Doctors usually treat sore throats with antibiotics if there is the slightest doubt of these complications occurring.

Can an acute sore throat be treated only by Homeopathy—without antibiotics? The answer is *yes, if the correct treatment is chosen.* If the above treatment recommendations correspond *exactly* to your sore throat, don't hesitate to follow them, but the symptoms should then disappear less than 24 hours later. If you're not certain of the treatment choice, or if it has no effect, check with your homeopathic physician who will attempt to find the treatment which most closely corresponds to your symptoms.

If he cannot find enough characteristic symptoms to safely prescribe a homeopathic treatment, he may prescribe an antibiotic rather than have you run a risk of sore throat complications. Don't be surprised by this. For treating sore throats, however, the doctor must be right 100 % of the time; if the patient has to come back for a second consultation, complications may have already set in. If a homeopathic doctor prescribes antibiotics, it's because he or she has your best health interests in mind.

The homeopathic treatment for chronic sore throats.

Chronic sore throats are another problem. In Allopathy, there exists no terrain treatment so you should consult a homeopathic physician if you suffer two or three successive sore throats. Ask his or her advice even if the treatment outlined above for acute sore throat helps.

Should children who often suffer from sore throats have their tonsils removed?

Never! The long-term preventive homeopathic treatment should be sufficient. Moreover, the tonsils are not merely a couple of almond-shaped UFO's obstructing the throat, but rather an excellent system of defense against germs. They should be left in place. If they are taken out, the first barrier against germs is no longer there, so they spread further and faster. If a child has very large tonsils, the best solution is to wait: as the child grows, the tonsils will remain the same size and take up less space in the throat.

▷ *Also see* **Pharyngitis (Sore throat).**

Spa cures

Spa cures are excellent supplements to homeopathic treatment because of their positive natural effects on the body's metabolism.

Spasms

- of the throat:
  IGNATIA AMARA 9 C.
  three pellets three times a day.
- of the stomach:
  NUX VOMICA 9 C.
  same dosage.
- of the muscles:
  BELLADONNA 9 C.
  same dosage.
- of the eyelids: *see* this entry.

- *Also see* **Breath-holding spell, Hyperventilation, Vaginismus.**

Specific

In Homeopathy, there is no remedy that is specific to a given disease. This means that no homeopathic medicine will automatically act just because the diagnosis of the disease is known. The treatment must always be selected according to the *symptoms* that are *characteristic* of each individual person.

Spigelia anthelmia

Base substance: Pink root or (annual) Worm grass.

Characteristic signs and symptoms:
Facial neuralgia, particularly on the left side; left-sided migraine; pain in the eyes; strong palpitations; intestinal pains.

Main clinical uses:
Facial neuralgia; pain caused by glaucoma: *WARNING - These diseases are serious. Contact your physician immediately for treatment recommendation.*
Migraines; peristaltic disorders caused by worms.

Spinal column

If joint pain is localized in the spinal column, you may supplement the treatment outlined under the heading, **Rheumatism** with one of the following remedies. Take three pellets three times a day.

Neck:
LACHNANTHES TINCTORIA 9 C.

Back (from the base of the neck to the waist):
- for the upper part of the back,
  CIMICIFUGA RACEMOSA 9 C.
- for the lower part,
  SULPHUR 9 C.

Lumbar region:
- lumbago with pains radiating to the chest,
  BERBERIS VULGARIS 9 C.
- lumbago with pains that are made worse by the least movement, or by coughing,
  BRYONIA ALBA 9 C.

- lumbago that is relieved by movement or by lying on a hard surface,
  RHUS TOXICODENDRON 9 C.
- lumbago with muscle cramps,
  NUX VOMICA 9 C.

Sacrum:
AESCULUS HIPPOCASTANUM 9 C.

Coccyx:
HYPERICUM PERFORATUM 9 C.

Spleen

WARNING: You must check with your physician.
Some diseases of the spleen may be treated by Homeopathy. You may begin taking the following remedy, whatever the symptoms:
HELIANTHUS ANNUS 5 C,
three pellets three times a day.

Spoiled Food

Eating spoiled food can cause vomiting and diarrhea, which are very unpleasant but not usually life-threatening.
Take:
ARSENICUM ALBUM 9 C,
PYROGENIUM 9 C,
alternate three pellets of each, three times a day for three days.

Spongia tosta

Base substance: Toasted sponge.

Characteristic signs and symptoms:
A sensation of dryness of the oral mucosa; barking cough, relieved by eating and drinking; sensation of suffocation due to anxiety with palpitations; enlarged, indurated thyroid gland; indurated testicles.

Main clinical uses:
Laryngitis with stridor; asthma; hard goiter; pancreatitis.

Even for slight falls, use ARNICA right away.

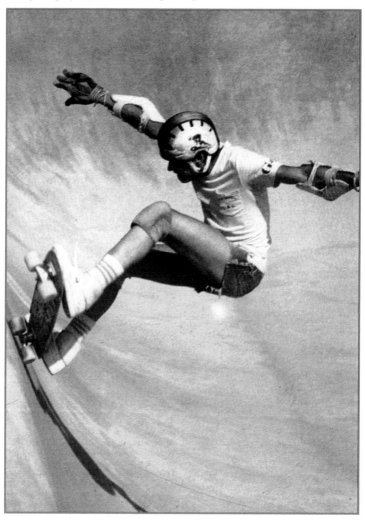

Sports

Preparing for sports:
Take three pellets of one or more of the following remedies three times a day, beginning several days before the sports activity or competition begins. This technique does not in any manner constitute artificial stimulation or doping.

ARNICA MONTANA 9 C,
prepares the body for making an effort.

GELSEMIUM SEMPERVIRENS 9 C,
alleviates the nervous fright of anticipation.

In case of complications:
- for muscle cramps,
  NUX VOMICA 9 C,
  three pellets three times a day.
- for fatigue due to excessive muscle strain, stiffness or epicondylitis,
  RHUS TOXICODENDRON 9 C,
  same dosage.

In case of injuries, ▷ *see* this entry.

Even for slight falls, use ARNICA right away to prevent bruising and complications.

Spots in front of the eyes, ▷ *see* **Eyes.**

Sprains

A simple sprain can be successfully treated by Homeopathy. Only a physician can tell how bad a sprain might be though, so you should consult a doctor for any sprain that causes real pain. The treatment given below can treat minor sprains.

General treatment for sprains:
ARNICA MONTANA 9 C,
RHUS TOXICODENDRON 9 C,
RUTA GRAVEOLENS 9 C,
alternate three pellets of each, three times a day.

Local treatment:
RUTA GRAVEOLENS M.T.,
twenty-five drops onto a compress applied three times a day.

Treatment for tendency to repeated sprains:
NATRUM CARBONICUM 9 C,
three pellets three times a day, for two weeks a month over several months.

Stannum metallicum

Base substance: Tin.

Characteristic signs and symptoms:
A feeling of weakness in the chest, making it impossible to speak; sweet tasting saliva; coughing when speaking, laughing or singing; exhausting nocturnal sweating.

Main clinical uses:
Chronic bronchitis; dilation of the bronchial passages.

Staphysagria

Base substance: the Palmated Larkspur seeds, also known as Louse seeds.

Characteristic signs and symptoms:
Poorly concealed irritability; constant sexual thoughts; emotional oversensitivity; decayed teeth; burning pains in the urethra, relieved by urinating; warts; styes; wounds caused by a sharp instrument.

Main clinical uses:
Nervous cystitis; styes: *WARNING - These diseases are serious. You must contact your physician immediately for treatment recommendation.*
Neuralgia; warts; healing of surgical operations.

Sterility (as in childbearing)

The causes of sterility are usually **organic** and require medical or surgical treatment. Homeopathy can only treat the psychological causes of infertility. Check with a homeopathic physician (a gynecologist, if possible).

▷ *See* **Organic diseases.**

Sticta pulmonaria

Base substance: Lungmoss.

Characteristic signs and symptoms: Stopped-up, dry nose with constant need to blow the nose; pain or pressure at the base of the nose; dry cough, worse at night; alternating joint pains and coryza.

Main clinical uses: Cough with measles: *WARNING - This condition is serious. You should consult your physician for advice.* Acute, dry coryza; frontal sinusitis following coryza.

Stiffness

Due to fatigue: ARNICA MONTANA 9 C, RHUS TOXICODENDRON 9 C, alternate three pellets of each, three times a day.

▷ *See* **Sports.**

During a spike of fever: PYROGENIUM 9 C, RHUS TOXICODENDRON 9 C, alternate three pellets of each, three times a day.

'Stitch in the side'

If you have a stitch (sharp little pain) in your side, try the following: first,

put your feet together, bend forward without bending your knees, pick up a pebble (or pretend to), stand up straight, bend again and put the pebble back, and stand up straight again. The stitch should have disappeared. You may also take: CEANOTHUS AMERICANUS 5 C, three pellets when pain occurs. Repeat two minutes later if necessary.

Stomach

For abdominal pains: *WARNING: Abdominal pains should be carefully examined by a doctor.* You may try taking three pellets of one of the following remedies at a rate of every hour or three times a day, *but if you don't obtain quick relief, get to a doctor.*

• if the belly feels warm and hurts when it is pressed on: *Get to a doctor immediately.*
• if you have a mild "stitch" in your side, CEANOTHUS AMERICANUS 9 C.
• for abdominal pains that are relieved by doubling or curling up in bed: *Contact a doctor immediately.*
• for abdominal pains occurring after being angry or upset, COLOCYNTHIS 9 C.
• sensation of belly cramps, CUPRUM METALLICUM 9 C.
• abdominal pain that is relieved by standing up straight or bending over backward, DIOSCOREA VILLOSA 9 C.
• abdominal pains after being sad or irritated, IGNATIA AMARA 9 C.
• pains relieved by pressure of the hand on the abdomen, MAGNESIA PHOSPHORICA 9 C.

• pains relieved by heat on the abdomen,
  MAGNESIA PHOSPHORICA 9 C.
• abdominal pains during menstrual periods,
  MAGNESIA PHOSPHORICA 9 C.
• abdominal pains during pregnancy:
You must see a doctor.

REMEMBER: Anytime you or a member of your family have true abdominal pain (not indigestion, upset stomach, etc.), you must be examined by a doctor as soon as possible (even at night). Call your physician or hospital emergency room.

▷ *Also see* **Colic, Diarrhea.**

Acidic stomach, "heartburn":
  IRIS VERSICOLOR 9 C,
  SULPHURICUM ACIDUM 9 C,
  alternate three pellets of each,
  three times a day.

Burning sensations in the stomach:
(Take three pellets three times a day.)
• with thirst for small, frequently-repeated drinks of cold water,
  ARSENICUM ALBUM 9 C.
• with thirst, but even the smallest drink of liquid makes pain worse,
  CANTHARIS 9 C.
• not only in the stomach but throughout the entire digestive tract,
  IRIS VERSICOLOR 9 C.
• with thirst for large quantities of cold water,
  PHOSPHORUS 9 C.

Stomach cramps:
• relieved by burping,
  CARBO VEGETABILIS 9 C.
• relieved by external warmth or heat,
  MAGNESIA PHOSPHORICA 9 C.
• stomach is sensitive to pressure,
  NUX VOMICA 9 C.
• relieved by a short nap,
  NUX VOMICA 9 C.

Pain: ▷ *see* this entry.
Consult the paragraphs within entitled "Acidic stomach," "Burning

sensations," "Stomach cramps," "Heaviness after meals."

Gastric disorders:
▷ *see* **Digestion.**

Gastritis:
▷ *see* the paragraphs "Acidic stomach," "Burning sensations," "Stomach cramps."

Hiatal hernia:
▷ *see* **Hernia.**

Indigestion:
▷ *see* **Digestion.**

Heaviness after meals:
  NUX VOMICA 9 C.

Stomach or duodenal ulcer: (See your doctor.)
  ARGENTUM NITRICUM 9 C,
  KALI BICHROMICUM 9 C,
  alternate three pellets of each,
  three times a day during episodes of pain.

▷ *Also see* **Bloatedness, Drowsiness, Eructation, Hiccups, Nausea, Vomiting.**

Stomatitis

▷ *See* **Mouth.**

Storms

A general feeling of uneasiness when a storm is approaching:
  RHODODENDRON
  CHRYSANTHEMUM 9 C.
  three pellets every half hour.

Fear of storms:
  PHOSPHORUS 9 C.
  same dosage.

Strabismus (squint)

Strabismus cannot be corrected by
Homeopathy, and must be treated by
an eye doctor (ophthalmologist).
If you had strabismus as a child, tell
your homeopathic doctor; he or she
will take it into account when
establishing your terrain treatment.

In case of strabismus that develops
during the course of a fever, take:
GELSEMIUM SEMPERVIRENS 9 C,
three pellets three times a day.

Stramonium

Base substance: Thorn apple or
Jimsonweed.

Characteristic signs and symptoms:
Nightmares with fear of the dark and
being alone; stuttering; restlessness
with a tendency to bite others;
bumping the head against a wall
causes no apparent discomfort.

Main clinical uses:
Nightmares; stuttering; moody, restless
children; measles that are slow
(reluctant) to break out.

Strangulated hernia

▷ *See* **Hernia.**

Strophanthus hispidus

Base substance: the seeds of
Strophanthus (Onage).

Main clinical use:
Nervous heart, characteristic of
smokers and drinkers.

Stuttering

There is no harm in trying this
remedy, but you are advised to consult
a homeopathic physician who can
determine a long-term treatment
course. Deep-seated stuttering is
difficult to get rid of.
STRAMONIUM 9 C,
three pellets three times a day.

Styes

Styes are small, inflamed cysts on the
edge of an eyelid.

General treatment:
HEPAR SULPHURIS CALCAREUM 9 C,
PULSATILLA 9 C,
alternate three pellets of each,
three times a day.

Local treatment:
Apply CALENDULA ointment locally
twice a day.

_WARNING: If symptoms worsen or
persist for more than 72 hours,
discontinue use of the above medicines
and consult your doctor._

Sugar in the urine

▷ *See* **Diabetes, Urine test.**

Suicide (Thoughts of)

▷ *See* **Depression.**

Sulphur

Base substance: Sulfur.

Suitable for:
Jovial, optimistic people who tend to
overphilosophize. They often have
congestive, ruddy complexions and are
negligent of the way they dress.

Characteristic signs and symptoms:
Red, burning, itchy rashes that are
made worse by water; tendency to
mucus secretions (colds, bronchitis,
diarrhea, etc.) and to effusions
(pleurisy, synovitis); a craving for fats,
alcohol and sugar; excess body heat; a
sensation of localized cutaneous
congestion, particularly on the sole of
the foot (the person must take off his
or her shoes for relief); alternation of
the above disorders; general
aggravation of symptoms by exposure
to heat and being in a standing
position, relief by being outside.

Main clinical uses:
Flu-like symptoms; eczema; diarrhea;
allergy; migraine; rheumatism;
effusions; menopause; chronic
alcoholism.

<u>WARNING:</u> *If condition worsens or
persists for more than 72 hours, check
with your physician.*

Sulphuricum acidum

Base substance: Sulfuric acid.

Suitable for: The complications of
excess drinking.

Characteristic signs and symptoms:
A sensation of trembling on the inside;
bleeding of dark blood; fever blisters; a
feeling of emptiness in the stomach,
relieved by drinking alcohol.

Main clinical uses:
Excess drinking: <u>WARNING</u> - *This
disease is serious. You should consult
your physician for advice.*
Fever blisters; stomatitis; bleeding.

Sun

Repeated exposure to the sun
prematurely ages the skin. Don't forget
that tanning is a defensive reaction of

the body to protect itself from the
negative effects of the ultraviolet rays
contained in sunlight. If you overdo it,
there is even a risk of skin cancer.
Sunlight is essential to life, but you
should expose yourself to it slowly and
cautiously.

Allergy to the sun:
● in case of hives from exposure to the
sun,
APIS MELLIFICA 9 C,
three pellets three times a day.

Sunburn:
● for red, painful skin,
BELLADONNA 9 C,
three pellets three times a day.
● in case of burns with blistering, or
peeling away of the upper layer of
skin,
CANTHARIS 9 C,
same dosage.

*Sunstroke, fainting due to the heat of
the sun:* <u>WARNING</u> - *Head for
immediate medical care.*

For aftereffects, take:
GLONOINUM 9 C,
three pellets, every five to fifteen
minutes, depending on seriousness.

Prevention:
NATRUM MURIATICUM 9 C,
is the best preventive remedy for
people whose skin cannot stand
the sun. Take three pellets three
times a day, beginning two weeks
before you are exposed to the sun.
Continue the treatment throughout
the exposure period.

Suppressing a disease

When a disease is treated by
considering only those symptoms
involving the affected organ, without
taking the patient's general condition
into account, the *cure* thus obtained is
a *suppression.* The local symptoms are

215

suppressed but they come back again, like the legendary hydra (many-headed serpent) of Lerne whose heads grew back as soon as they were cut off. An example of this is a cortisone-based ointment which will *suppress* eczema rather than cure it. When the ointment is stopped, the eczema returns. The principle is the same for sclerosing treatments for hemorrhoids and varicose veins. Suppressing sweating, even heavy sweating, with strong chemical anti-perspirants is also needlessly harsh; sweating is a natural protective mechanism.

Suppuration

▷ *See* **Abscess.**

Surgery

Homeopathic physicians are not opposed to surgery—when it is needed. Homeopathic doctors do, however, probably recommend surgery less often than their surgeon counterparts. If a health problem is a benign one (uncomplicated gallstones or uterine fibroma, for example), and the patient is not suffering, homeopaths prefer to first try a homeopathic treatment.

To prepare for surgery, take:
GELSEMIUM SEMPERVIRENS 12 C, one unit-dose tube on the first day, ARNICA MONTANA 12 C, one unit-dose tube on the second day, NUX VOMICA 12 C, one unit-dose tube on the third day. Continue this treatment course in three-day cycles (GELSEMIUM SEMPERVIRENS 12 C, ARNICA MONTANA 12 C, NUX VOMICA 12 C) changing

remedies every day. Begin a week before the operation and continue taking it for a week afterward (once you're allowed to take medicine by mouth).
If you do this correctly, your surgeon may pay you the compliment of being the "best patient in the ward."

If you haven't followed this treatment and complications develop, take three pellets of one of the following remedies three times a day after you're allowed to take medicine by mouth.

• for nerve pain (in a stump, for example),
ALLIUM CEPA 9 C.
• retention of urine,
CAUSTICUM 9 C.
• post-operative vomiting,
PHOSPHORUS 9 C.
• bloating in the abdomen,
RAPHANUS SATIVUS 9 C.
• abdominal pain,
STAPHYSAGRIA 9 C.
• if the scar takes a long time to heal,
STAPHYSAGRIA 9 C.

▷ *Also see* **Cosmetic surgery.**

Swallowing (Difficulty in)

If swallowing is impossible:
WARNING - See your doctor.
HYOSCYAMUS NIGER 9 C, three pellets three times a day.

If you don't seem to be able to stop swallowing:
LACHESIS 9 C, three pellets three times a day.

Sweating

▷ *See* **Perspiration.**

Swelling

▷ *See* **Edema.**

Sympathetic nervous system

Damage to the sympathetic nervous system may be treated by Homeopathy. The symptoms are variable. Check with a doctor.

Symphytum officinale

Base substance: Comfrey.

Main clinical uses:
Trauma to the bones with slow healing of fractures; trauma to the eyes.

Symptom

For a homeopathic physician, a symptom[1] is an integral part of the general concept of the patient, disease, and treatment. A symptom is the expression of the patient's reactional mode—an attempt on the part of the body to eliminate the disease.
The physician must take into account all of the patient's symptoms when diagnosing and prescribing a remedy capable of effecting a cure (see **Reactional Mode**).

---

1. **Signs and symptoms:**
- a sign is something measurable or observable (your temperature or blood pressure, for example); it is characteristic of the disease being diagnosed; a sign is objective.
- a symptom is something that the patient describes about his ailment (pain, dizziness, nausea, etc. are symptoms); a symptom is characteristic of a given patient and how he or she feels; it is subjective.
For example: 'Tenderness' when the doctor pushes down on Johnny's lower right abdomen is a **sign** of appendicitis; the pain felt at that moment by Johnny is a **symptom.** A normal, non-painful abdomen is called a "non-tender belly" in clinical terminology (based on clinical observation).

The best doctors in any field say that making a diagnosis depends heavily on listening to what patients have to say about their ailments *(symptoms)*. A medical doctor trained in Homeopathy is particularly aware of the importance of the symptoms a patient describes when discussing his or her problem. A correct diagnosis can only be made by careful listening. Good homeopathic medicine means being more interested in treating a person and his or her problem than in just observing and treating a particular type of disease. Symptoms are of primordial importance in Homeopathy.

Symptomatic treatment

Medically speaking, a "symptomatic treatment" is one which aims to alleviate the symptoms of the disease rather than its cause. For example, when you take aspirin to stop a headache (symptom), you are undergoing a symptomatic treatment.

The advice given in *The Guide* is mainly symptomatic, and primarily applicable to *acute illnesses.* If a disorder continues, reappears after an apparent cure, or even becomes a recurrent illness (migraine, asthma, etc.), you should consult a homeopathic physician. He or she can prescribe a terrain treatment (see **Terrain**).

Synovitis, effusion of synovia

Inflammation of a joint lining, often with accompanying fluid build-up ("water on a joint," "water on the knee," etc.). The origin is frequently

arthritic or tra matic. The joint is
swollen and painful.
Take three pellets of one or more of
the following remedies.

Depending on the cause:
- inflammation of the joint,
  APIS MELLIFICA 9 C.
- after injury,
  ARNICA MONTANA 9 C.

Depending on the circumstances:
Pain relieved:
- by exposure to cold,
  APIS MELLIFICA 9 C.
- by resting,
  BRYONIA ALBA 9 C.
- by external pressure,
  BRYONIA ALBA 9 C.
- by motion of the joint,
  KALI IODATUM 9 C.

Pain aggravated:
- by pressure,
  APIS MELLIFICA 9 C.
- at night,
  KALI IODATUM 9 C.

For chronic cases:
  CALCAREA FLUORICA 9 C.

Syphilis

Syphilis cannot be treated
homeopathically; it must be treated by
pharmaceuticals and according to
clinical and biological guidelines.
Nonetheless, you should also consult a
homeopathic physician if you have
been diagnosed as having syphilis in
order to receive a terrain treatment
that will help to prevent the
consequences of the disease.

TU

Healthy, beautiful teeth with good homeopathic care.

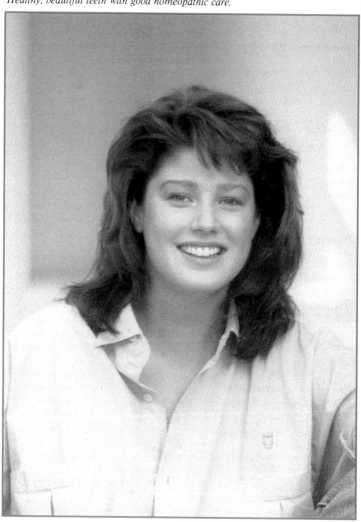

Tabacum

Base substance: the fresh plant of Tobacco.

Characteristic signs and symptoms: Cold sweats; paleness; dizziness on opening the eyes; nausea; excess salivation; a feeling of emptiness in the pit of the stomach; a craving for fresh air; a need to keep the chest uncovered.

Main clinical uses: Vomiting during pregnancy: _WARNING - As with any medication, if you are pregnant or nursing a baby, you must have professional advice._ Travel or motion sickness.

Taenia (Tapeworm)

▷ See **Worms (Intestinal).**

Tailbone

▷ See **Coccyx.**

Taraxacum officinale

Base substance: the Dandelion.

Characteristic signs and symptoms: "Map-like tongue," sensitive to the touch; bitter taste in the mouth; enlarged liver; yellow skin; migraine.

Main clinical uses: Jaundice; hepatic insufficiency: _WARNING - These diseases are serious. Contact your physician immediately for treatment recommendation._ Migraine headaches.

Tarentula cubensis

Base substance: Cuban tarantula.

Main clinical use: Anthrax infections: _WARNING - This disease is serious. Contact your physician immediately for treatment recommendation._

Tarentula hispana

Base substance: the Tarantula.

Characteristic signs and symptoms: Nervous restlessness, relieved by music, aggravated by being watched or touched; convulsions; constantly moving head.

Main clinical uses: Restless children.

Taste in the mouth (Bad)

▷ See **Mouth.**

Teeth

WARNING: If conditions persist, discontinue use of the following remedies and consult your dentist or doctor.

Abscess:
MERCURIUS SOLUBILIS 9 C, three pellets three times a day.

Tooth decay:
• if decayed teeth are black, CREOSOTUM 9 C, three pellets three times a day.
• if decayed teeth are gray, MERCURIUS SOLUBILIS 9 C, three pellets three times a day.

Loosening of teeth:
LYCOPODIUM CLAVATUM 9 C, MERCURIUS SOLUBILIS 9 C, alternate three pellets of each, three times a day, two weeks per

month over a period of several months.

Teething: ▷ *see* **Dentition.**

Painful teeth (toothache):
Three pellets of one of the following remedies three times a day.
● for toothache relieved by warm water,
    ARSENICUM ALBUM 9 C.
● for very sharp, unbearable pains,
    CHAMOMILLA 9 C.
● for pains which become worse when speaking,
    CHAMOMILLA 9 C.
● for pains relieved by cold water,
    COFFEA CRUDA 9 C.
● for pains relieved by rubbing the cheeks,
    MERCURIUS SOLUBILIS 9 C.
● for toothaches during menstrual periods,
    STAPHYSAGRIA 9 C.

For local relief of toothache, put a few drops of:
    PLANTAGO MAJOR M. T.,
    onto the gums around the painful tooth.

Tooth enamel (loss of):
    CALCAREA FLUORICA 9 C,
    three pellets three times a day, twenty days a month over a period of several months. This treatment should help halt the further loss of tooth enamel.

Tooth extraction (before having a tooth pulled):
    ARNICA MONTANA 9 C,
    GELSEMIUM SEMPERVIRENS 9 C,
    alternate three pellets of each, three times a day beginning the day before your tooth is to be pulled.

Fistula around the teeth:
    MERCURIUS SOLUBILIS 9 C,
    SILICEA 9 C,
    alternate three pellets of each, three times a day. See your dentist immediately.

Gum fluxion (swelling):
    MERCURIUS SOLUBILIS 9 C,
    three pellets three times a day. See your dentist immediately.

Shape of teeth:
▷ *see* **Typology.**

Grinding and gritting of the teeth:
    BELLADONNA 9 C,
    three pellets three times a day.

Nerve pain in a tooth:
    BELLADONNA 9 C,
    three pellets three times a day.

Preparing for dental work:
▷ *see above,* "Tooth extraction."

Wisdom tooth:
For pain caused by incoming wisdom teeth,
    CHEIRIANTHUS 9 C,
    three pellets three times a day.

Telephone

Homeopathic physicians often give advice over the phone, particularly when they know the patient well, and the illness is a benign one.
Before you call your doctor:
- be sure to have paper and a pencil handy as the names of homeopathic medicines are difficult to remember.
- have your latest prescription in front of you.
- if you have a fever, take your temperature first and write it down.
- learn how to describe your own symptoms—note what triggered the ailment, and under what circumstances it is made better or worse (by exposure to cold, to heat, in a specific position, by eating or drinking something in particular, etc.). The more details you can give, the better your physician will be able to help you.

Tendinitis

The inflammation of a tendon,
generally following exertion.
Take:
  RHUS TOXICODENDRON 9 C,
  three pellets three times a day.

A local treatment may be useful;
consult your homeopathic physician.

Tennis elbow

▷ *See* **Epicondylitis.**

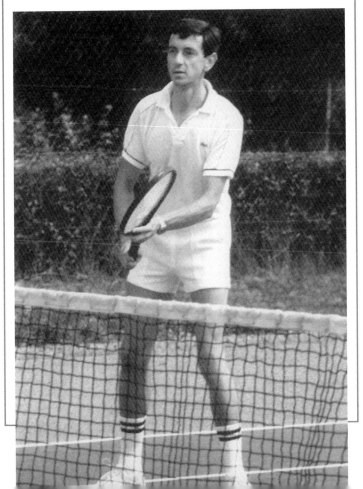

Terebinthina

Base substance: Turpentine oil.

Characteristic signs and symptoms:
Cystitis with dark brown urine that smells like violets; burning pains in the kidney region; various types of bleeding.

Main clinical uses:
Cystitis; pyelonephritis: <u>WARNING</u> - *These diseases are serious. You must consult your physician immediately for treatment recommendation.*

Terrain (Constitution)

The idea of *terrain* in medicine isn't new; it is once again receiving the importance it deserves as immunology makes everyone aware of how important the body's natural defenses are in fighting off disease.

According to the concept of terrain, a microorganism (bacteria, parasites, or even a sub-microorganism, like a virus) is much less potentially harmful to you if your body is healthy and prepared to ward it off. A microorganism becomes invasive when it is allowed to, when the body's natural defenses are weak—when the *terrain* is right for the invader to gain a foothold. The microorganism is severely handicapped if it can't find the "fertile soil" it needs to grow in and do its damage.

Homeopathy concentrates on reinforcing your body's own resistance to germs, or preparing your *terrain* defenses so that invasive microorganisms cannot set in and cause disease. A long-term treatment is the best way to maintain a healthy terrain condition because it is a systematic and in-depth approach to your preventive health needs. Because a long-term treatment is an in-depth treatment program that depends on your total array of symptoms, you should consult a homeopathic doctor. An individualized long-term treatment for any ailment is one that a trained homeopath should prescribe for you.

Testicles

Undescended testicles:
If you have a male child with this condition, he needs to be examined by a doctor.
You may try:
> AURUM METALLICUM 9 C,
> three pellets three times a day, twenty days a month over a period of three months, but the child must be seen by a doctor in any case.

Painful testicles:
> HAMAMELIS VIRGINICA 9 C,
> three pellets three times a day.

Eczema of the scrotum:
> CROTON TIGLIUM 9 C,
> three pellets three times a day.

Swollen testicles:
> PULSATILLA 9 C,
> three pellets three times a day.

Herpes of the scrotum:
> MERCURIUS SOLUBILIS 9 C,
> three pellets three times a day.

Hydrocele (watery cyst around a testicle):
> RHODODENDRON CHRYSANTHEMUM 9 C,
> three pellets three times a day.

Orchitis (inflammation of the testicles):
▷ *see above* "Swollen testicles."

Pain to touch:
> SPONGIA TOSTA 9 C,
> three pellets three times a day.

WARNING: You may take the above remedies but a doctor should be told about any problems with the testicles (even if the problem goes away first).

Tetanus

WARNING: _You must be seen by a doctor._
Prevention is the best treatment—make sure that you and your children are immunized.
REMEMBER: Keep your immunizations up-to-date.

If you are cut, ask your doctor if you need a booster. The treatment of someone who has tetanus (a very serious disease involving paralysis) must always be done in a hospital. The following homeopathic medicines can be given along with _(never instead of)_ the standard medical treatment:
CICUTA VIROSA 9 C,
HYPERICUM PERFORATUM 9 C,
LEDUM PALUSTRE 9 C,
dissolve ten pellets of each in a large glass of water and give one teaspoonful every hour, beginning as soon as possible.

Tetany

▷ _See_ **Hyperventilation.**

Teucrium marum verum

Base substance: Cat thyme.

Characteristic signs and symptoms:
Polyps in the nose; anal pruritus.

Main clinical uses:
Verminosis (intestinal worms):
WARNING - This disease is serious. Contact your physician immediately for treatment recommendation.
Atrophic rhinitis; polyps in the nose.

Theridion curassavicum

Base substance: the Theridion, a Black spider from Curaçoa Island.

Characteristic signs and symptoms:
Sensitivity to noise—the slightest noise seems to penetrate clear to the teeth; dizziness aggravated by closing the eyes.

Main clinical uses:
Sensitivity to noise; dizziness; migraines.

Thinness

There is no short-term homeopathic treatment for excessive thinness. Check with a homeopathic physician for a long-term treatment (this will be the best way to evaluate and treat this problem).

Thlaspi bursa pastoris

Base substance: the Shepherd's purse.

Main clinical use:
Heavy menstrual bleeding every other month.

Throat

For treatment of throat ailments, _see_ the entries which seem most appropriate: **Sore throat, Pharyngitis,** etc.

Thrush

▷ _See_ **Candidiasis.**

Thuja occidentalis

Base substance: the Tree of life or White cedar.

Suitable for:
Water retention in certain tissues,

particularly in the hips of women; perspiration from uncovered areas of the body; the side-effects of vaccinations.

Characteristic signs and symptoms:
Slowing down of psychic processes; intellectual slowness; emotional sensitivity (music makes the patient cry); body sensations which could not possibly be real—something "alive" in the stomach, a feeling as if the bones were made of glass; migraine that feels as if nails were being hammered into the head; colds with green mucus secretions; wet, soft warts; enlarged prostate gland; fibroma; general aggravation of symptoms by exposure to humidity.

Main clinical uses:
Warts; polyps; rheumatism; periodontitis; diarrhea; chronic coryza (rhinitis and head colds).

Thyroid gland

Disorders of the thyroid gland may respond to homeopathic treatment but must be evaluated by a doctor. *Early Grave's disease (hyperthyroidism)* is frequently within the scope of Homeopathy. *Hypothyroidism* should always be treated with a classical hormonal treatment or as your doctor advises. It is essential to know the cause of any goiter—check with your doctor or a specialist in endocrinology. Cysts of the thyroid gland do not respond to Homeopathy. Again, you cannot heal thyroid disorders by yourself—check with your doctor.

Tics (from nervousness)

Don't scold your child for having nervous tics—he or she would probably be just as glad to get rid of them. Instead, take the child to a homeopathic physician, who can propose a treatment plan to help them go away.
In the meantime, give:
AGARICUS MUSCARIUS 9 C,
NATRUM MURIATICUM 9 C,
alternate three pellets of each, three times a day until your appointment with the homeopath.

Tongue

The appearance of the tongue frequently helps the homeopathic physician to choose the appropriate remedies and may be an important clue to what is going on elsewhere in the body.

Coated tongue:
Take three pellets of one of the indicated remedies three times a day.
● tongue coated with a whitish film that looks like the skin of milk,
ANTIMONIUM CRUDUM 9 C.
● black tongue,
CARBO VEGETABILIS 9 C.
● yellow tongue,
HYDRASTIS CANADENSIS 9 C.
● tongue coated only at the back,
NUX VOMICA 9 C.
● a red triangle at the tip of the tongue,
RHUS TOXICODENDRON 9 C.
● "map-like or geographical" tongue (normal bumps surrounded by patches of coated bumps; these patches may migrate or come together, producing a map-like appearance),
TARAXACUM OFFICINALE 9 C.

Swollen tongue (If a swollen tongue affects breathing, contact a doctor immediately):
Same dosage.
● if the tongue seems swollen and is difficult to move, if it trembles,
GELSEMIUM SEMPERVIRENS 9 C.

• tongue is actually swollen, the edge shows the imprint of the teeth,
MERCURIUS SOLUBILIS 9 C.

Burning tongue:
Same dosage.
• burning pains from drinking a hot liquid,
CANTHARIS 9 C.
• burning pains in the tongue without apparent cause,
IRIS VERSICOLOR 9 C.
If you frequently experience a burning sensation on your tongue, check with your dentist to see if two different kinds of metal were used in your fillings or appliances. If so, you may be feeling a tiny discharge set off between the metals.

Tonsils, Tonsillitis

▷ *See* **Sore throat.**

Tracheitis (Tracheal cold)

Inflammation of the trachea, characterized principally by coughing.

▷ *See* **Coughing.**

Tranquilizers

▷ *See* **Anxiety, Nervousness, Depression.**

Trauma (Minor)

Depending on the location of injury, take three pellets of one of the following remedies three times a day to avoid complications.
This treatment may be used in association with therapy in a hospital. If you have any questions as to the severity of an injury, see your doctor.

Head:
NATRUM SULPHURICUM 9 C.
WARNING: A doctor should know about any head trauma, even minor trauma. If a person gets sleepy after a bump or injury to the head, get him or her to a doctor. Children are especially prone to head injuries and should be seen by a doctor if they receive a blow to the skull.

Spinal cord: (See a doctor.)
HYPERICUM PERFORATUM 9 C.

Nerves (damaged): (See a doctor.)
HYPERICUM PERFORATUM 9 C.

Eyes: (See a doctor or eye doctor.)
• if there are bruises around the eyes,
LEDUM PALUSTRE 9 C.
• if there are no bruises,
SYMPHYTUM OFFICINALE 9 C.

Soft tissues (skin, muscles):
ARNICA MONTANA 9 C.

Breasts:
BELLIS PERENNIS 9 C.

▷ *Also see* **Injuries, Fractures.**

Traveling (Homeopathy and)

Preparing for a trip:
ARGENTUM NITRICUM 9 C,
three pellets three times a day.
Begin several days beforehand if you're afraid of traveling by car or plane.

▷ *Also see* **Vaccines.**

While traveling:
▷ *See below,* **Travel sickness.**

During your stay:
If you have trouble adapting to a local climate, take three pellets of one of the following remedies three times a day throughout your stay:
• in a hot country,
ANTIMONIUM CRUDUM 9 C.
• in humid areas,
DULCAMARA 9 C.

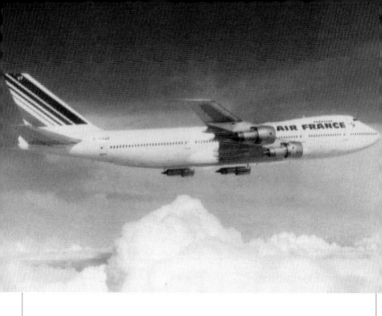

• intolerance to a maritime climate,
  NATRUM MURIATICUM 9 C.
Take *The Guide* with you on a trip so you can treat health problems while traveling.

Travel sickness
(Motion sickness)

Whatever the symptoms (nausea, vomiting, dizziness, an empty feeling, weakness) and whatever means of transport, take three pellets of one of the following remedies half an hour before leaving. Repeat dosage during the trip each time the symptoms recur.

Aggravated:
• by eating, moving the eyes, watching objects go by, exposure to fresh air (the person prefers to keep the windows rolled up),
  COCCULUS INDICUS 9 C.

• with cold sweats,
  PETROLEUM 9 C.

Improved:
• by eating,
  PETROLEUM 9 C.
• by exposure to fresh air (the patient rolls down the windows), by removing extra clothes, by closing eyes,
  TABACUM 9 C.

Trembling

Only trembling due to anxiety can be treated by Homeopathy.

▷ *See* **Anxiety, Nervousness (before an event).**

Treatment of Parkinson's disease is not within the scope of Homeopathy.

Trillium pendulum

Base substance: root of the Drooping trillium, also known as Wake Robin.

Characteristic signs and symptoms: Vaginal discharge of bright red blood, made worse by movement; dizziness and pains in the kidneys and thighs.

Main clinical uses: Uterine bleeding; bleeding from a uterine fibroma: *WARNING - These diseases are serious. You must consult your physician immediately for treatment recommendation.* Menopause; possible miscarriage.

Tropical diseases

These are often due to parasites and must be treated with chemical medicines to effect a cure. A homeopathic treatment may, nevertheless, be useful for the symptoms of tropical illnesses. Check with a doctor.

▷ *Also see* **Diarrhea, Malaria, Parasites.**

Tuberculinum

Base substance: Tuberculin.

Suitable for: People who catch cold easily.

Characteristic signs and symptoms: Inflammation of the mucous membranes; colds; diarrhea; cystitis; sore throat; bronchitis; a craving for air; alternation of above disorders.

Main clinical uses: Arterial hypotension (low blood pressure); the complications of tuberculosis: *WARNING - These diseases are serious. Contact your physician immediately for treatment recommendation.* Tendency to catch cold; acne; eczema; fatigue.

Tumors

Benign tumors may be treated homeopathically. Check with your doctor.

▷ *See* **Breasts, Warts.**

Malignant tumors are not within the scope of Homeopathy. Any tumor on your body must be examined by a physician.

▷ *See* **Cancer.**

Twitching of the eyes

▷ *See* **Eyelids.**

Typhoid Fever

A febrile (with fever) disease caused by Salmonella bacteria. Effective antibiotic medication to treat and cure typhoid fever is available and should be used. Follow your doctor's instructions. An accompanying homeopathic treatment may help to relieve some discomfort.

Typhoid Fever
(Paratyphoid fever)

Typhoid fever and paratyphoid fever are similar infectious diseases caused by different strains of Salmonella bacteria. Malaise, rash, fever, abdominal pain and swollen spleen are some usual signs. There may be

possible bowel and bleeding
complications if not diagnosed early
and treated with antibiotics.
Certain homeopathic medicines may
also be effective in the very early
stages. Must absolutely be seen by a
doctor.

Typology

A homeopathic doctor may sometimes
get a good idea of the homeopathic
treatment a person needs just by
seeing him or her in the waiting room,
before the consultation even begins.

Physical appearances alone are not
enough, of course, to make a final
diagnosis but they can often provide
important clues to the treatment a
person may need. These important
external clues, or profile, are part of
the patient's *typology*—his or her
external appearance and the diagnosis
impression it leaves.

Typology, to the observant physician,
can be very useful in orienting the
consultation in the right direction. The
doctor's questions, discussion with the
patient, and examination of the
patient will confirm (or refute) the
initial intuitive diagnosis.

Since typology is not an
experimentally established experience,
as applying the Law of Similars is, it is
not a wholly reliable method: it can
provide useful orientation but not
certitude.

Of course, a person's personality traits
will not be changed by any
homeopathic treatment—even the
appropriate one.

▷ *See* **Character.**

Ulcers

Duodenal or stomach ulcers:
▷ *see* **Stomach.**

Skin ulcers of the legs:

General treatment

(Three pellets of the selected remedy
or remedies three times a day.)

● skin ulcer that burns,
ARSENICUM ALBUM 9 C.
● with tendency to gangrene,
ARSENICUM ALBUM 9 C.
● with fever,
ARSENICUM ALBUM 9 C.
● after bruising of a vein,
BELLIS PERENNIS 9 C.
● with indurated edges,
CALCAREA FLUORICA 9 C.
● chronic skin ulcer that refuses to
heal, the skin around the ulcer is
bluish,
CARBO VEGETABILIS 9 C.
● foul-smelling skin ulcer,
HEPAR SULPHURIS CALCAREUM 9 C.
● with clean-cut edges,
KALI BICHROMICUM 9 C.
● the skin around the ulcer is purple,
LACHESIS 9 C.
● the ulcer is less painful when it
oozes,
LACHESIS 9 C.
● ulcer with irregular edges,
MERCURIUS SOLUBILIS 9 C.
● with stabbing pains,
NITRICUM ACIDUM 9 C.
● skin ulcer containing a mixture of
pus and blood,
PHOSPHORUS 9 C.

Local treatment

CLEMATIS VITALBA M.T.,
dissolve twenty-five drops in a
glass of lukewarm pre-boiled
water. Wash the ulcer with this
preparation once a day. Leave the
ulcer uncovered as much as
possible to expose it to the air and
sun; avoid ointments unless they
are required by your doctor.

Unicism

A number of homeopathic doctors give their patients only a single homeopathic remedy at a time. They feel that this should be sufficient to treat all of a patient's varied symptoms, and as symptoms change, they may change medicines, but one at a time.

This unicist approach depends on the doctor's training, the patient's collaboration and a correct understanding of the disease. There is no categorical position where unicism is concerned; most homeopathic doctors agree that one medicine alone should be used whenever possible. Some automatically practice unicism, while others tend to a reasonable pluralistic approach (use of several medicines, taken alternately).

Upset stomach

▷ See **Digestion.**

Urea, uremia

Uremia is an increase in a natural chemical, called urea, in the blood, but this is not a complete diagnosis. Sometimes the problem may be that the person is dehydrated, so the blood is more concentrated than normal (drinking more liquids might be the treatment).

In other cases, the causes are organic and must be diagnosed and treated by a doctor.

Treatment of uremia, to go along with your doctor's main treatment:
> UREA 5 C,
> three pellets three times a day.

Urethritis

Non-gonoccocal urethritis (gonorrhea is not the cause), will benefit from:
> PETROSELINUM SATIVUM 9 C,
> STAPHYSAGRIA 9 C,
> alternate three pellets of each, three times a day until the disorder disappears.

Check with your doctor if no improvement.

▷ Also see **Blennorrhagia.**

Uric acid

▷ See **Gout.**

Urinary infection

WARNING: If symptoms (burning urination, frequent urination, difficulty urinating, etc.) do not improve, check with your doctor. Anytime you notice blood in your urine, you should also be seen by a doctor.

Urinary infections may respond to Homeopathy, which can be effective both for acute and chronic cases of urinary and bladder infections.

With acute cases of cystitis (bladder infections), take:
> HEPAR SULPHURIS CALCAREUM 9 C,
> three pellets three times a day.

Supplement with:
> FORMICA RUFA 9 C,
> three pellets three times a day *for mild attacks;*
> CANTHARIS 9 C,
> three pellets three times a day *for severe attacks* (strong incessant pain, blood). See your doctor.

For false cystitis of nervous origin:
STAPHYSAGRIA 9 C,
three pellets three times a day.

For chronic cases:
Homeopathic physicians will often prescribe SEPIA, one of the basic homeopathic remedies used to treat urinary infection. If the patient has suffered from such an ailment for a long time, the treatment will last longer. To give an idea of what this entails, a person who has suffered from a chronic infection for twenty-five years may have to undergo a treatment lasting five years (without a homeopathic treatment he or she might continue to suffer attacks throughout their entire lifetime).

Urinating (Difficulty in), Dysuria

WARNING: Check with your doctor.

Depending on the symptoms, take three pellets of the selected remedy three times a day (or every hour for acute disorders).

Incessant urge to urinate but can't:
• of infectious origin,
MERCURIUS SOLUBILIS 9 C.
• of nervous origin,
STAPHYSAGRIA 9 C.

Urine comes out drop by drop:
CANTHARIS 9 C.

Patient is incapable of urinating in front of others (i.e., public toilets):
NATRUM MURIATICUM 9 C.

Involuntary passing of urine while coughing:
CAUSTICUM ANNUUM 9 C.
Consult your doctor if dysuria does not improve.

▷ *Also see* **Prostate gland disorders.**

Urine test

Should your urinalysis be abnormal (strongly positive for sugar, albumin, blood, bile salts and pigment, etc.), you should see a doctor. A precise diagnosis of the cause needs to be made.
The only thing for which you can treat yourself is the presence of phosphates in the urine (that turn it cloudy white). Take:
PHOSPHORICUM ACIDUM 9 C,
three pellets three times a day until cloudiness disappears.

▷ *Also see* **Diabetes.**

Urtica urens

Base substance: the small Stinging nettle.

Suitable for:
People who tend to have excessive amounts of uric acid in their blood.

Characteristic signs and symptoms:
Severe urticaria, aggravated by heat and water; cutaneous, burning sensation; vaginal itching.

Main clinical uses: Gout; urticaria; burning of the skin.

Urticaria (Hives)

A pink or red-colored eruption of itching wheals on the skin, occurring usually from systemic origin (hypersensitivity to certain foods or medicines, infection, psychic stimuli, etc.).
Take three pellets of one or more of the following remedies.

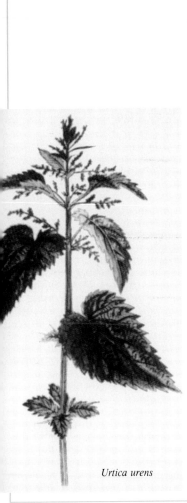

Urtica urens

Depending on the cause:
- urticaria caused by eating meat,
  ANTIMONIUM CRUDUM 9 C.
- urticaria at the seaside,
  ARSENICUM ALBUM 9 C.
- by eating crawfish,
  ASTACUS FLUVIATILUS 9 C.
- by drinking wine,
  CHLORALUM HYDRATE 9 C.
- by drinking milk,
  DULCAMARA 9 C.
- by eating strawberries,
  FRAGARIA VESCA 9 C.
- by eating lobster,
  HOMARUS 9 C.
- during menstrual periods,
  KALI CARBONICUM 9 C.
- due to the sun,
  NATRUM MURIATICUM 9 C.
- by eating pork,
  PULSATILLA 9 C.
- by eating seafood,
  URTICA URENS 9 C.
- after taking a bath,
  URTICA URENS 9 C.
- following strenuous exercise,
  URTICA URENS 9 C.

Depending on modifying circumstances:
Aggravated:
- at night,
  ARSENICUM ALBUM 9 C.
- by touching,
  URTICA URENS 9 C.

Improved:
- by cold water,
  APIS MELLIFICA 9 C.
- by hot water,
  ARSENICUM ALBUM 9 C.

Depending on the physical appearance:
- pinkish-looking urticaria,
  APIS MELLIFICA 9 C.
- reddish-looking urticaria,
  BELLADONNA 9 C.

Depending on the accompanying symptoms:
- urticaria with gastric discomfort,
  ANTIMONIUM CRUDUM 9 C.
- with Quincke's edema (flushed face, swollen lips due to allergic reaction),
  APIS MELLIFICA 9 C. (See your doctor.)

- with restlessness and anxiety,
  ARSENICUM ALBUM 9 C.
- with liver pain,
  ASTACUS FLUVIATILUS 9 C.
- with constipation,
  COPAIVA OFFICINALIS 9 C.
- with joint pain,
  URTICA URENS 9 C.

▷ *Also see* **Allergy.**

WARNING: Urticaria (hives) may be the sign of a serious disease or allergic reaction; if the patient looks ill, contact a doctor immediately.

Ustilago maidis

Base substance: Corn smut fungus.

Main clinical use:
Uterine bleeding, originating from a soft cervix: *WARNING - This disease is serious. Contact your physician immediately for treatment recommendation.*

Uterus

Fullness, awareness of having a uterus:
HELONIAS DIOICA 9 C,
three pellets three times a day.

Bleeding: Check with a doctor. If the flow is light and has occurred only recently, there are homeopathic treatments.

▷ *See* **Bleeding.**

Endometritis: You must be examined by a gynecologist.
Your doctor may prescribe:
HEPAR SULPHURIS CALCAREUM 9 C,
PYROGENIUM 9 C,
alternate three pellets of each, three times a day.

Heaviness in the lower pelvic area (a feeling of):
SEPIA 9 C,
three pellets three times a day.

Polyps:
check with a homeopathic physician.

Prolapsed organs: ▷ *see* **Prolapse.**

Menstrual periods: ▷ *see* this entry.

Uva ursi

Base substance: leaves of the red-berried trailing Arbutus, also known as Barberry.

Main clinical uses:
Chronic cystitis: *WARNING - This disease is serious. Contact your physician immediately for treatment recommendation.*

V W

Z

*"Homeopathy is a highly developed
health practice that uses
a systematic approach to the totality
of a person's health.
Anyone seeking a fuller understanding of health
and healing will find Homeopathy
extremely important and applicable."*

GAY GAER LUCE
(Ph.D., twice winner of the National Science Writers' Award)

Vaccines

Vaccines modify the **terrain** (see this entry). You or your child are more likely to experience the small annoyances of everyday existence for a while. This is not a reason for not being vaccinated, or opposing immunizations.

Tetanus is a disease which may be fatal; it is better to be vaccinated against it than to run a risk.

Poliomyelitis is also a dangerous disease; it is better to be vaccinated against it. Non-immunized women who are likely to become pregnant should be vaccinated against *rubella.*

Accept recommended vaccinations during an epidemic or whenever there is a major risk of contagion (such as a bad flu epidemic, especially if you fall into a risk category).

Generally speaking, examine the pros and cons: some vaccinations are mandatory, some are not (flu vaccine). Some may have rare but definite unwanted side-effects. Talk to your homeopathic physician.

In the evening following a vaccination, always take:
> THUJA OCCIDENTALIS 30 C,
> one unit-dose tube.

Should complications occur, take three pellets of the appropriate remedy three times a day and call your doctor.

Abscess:
> SILICEA 9 C.

Loss of weight:
> SILICEA 9 C.

Asthma:
> ANTIMONIUM TARTARICUM 9 C.

Diarrhea:
> THUJA OCCIDENTALIS 9 C.

General state of weakness:
- from an old vaccination,
  > SILICEA 9 C.

- from a recent vaccination,
  > THUJA OCCIDENTALIS 9 C.

Fever:
> ACONITUM NAPELLUS 9 C.

Lymph node swelling:
> SILICEA 9 C.

Recurring otitis (ear infections):
(Check with your doctor.)
> SILICEA 9 C.

Local skin reaction:
- swelling wheals,
  > APIS MELLIFICA 9 C.
- redness,
  > BELLADONNA 9 C.
- acute suppuration (recent pus),
  > MERCURIUS SOLUBILIS 9 C.
- crust or scab,
  > MEZEREUM 9 C.
- chronic suppuration (old onset of pus),
  > SILICEA 9 C.
- forming of a pustule or blister,
  > THUJA OCCIDENTALIS 9 C.

Recurring rhinopharyngitis:
> SILICEA 9 C.

Vaginal discharge (White)

WARNING: Check with your doctor.

White vaginal discharge is called *leukorrhea.* It is composed of mucus and pus (white cells). When the flow is not heavy and is unaccompanied by symptoms, it is "physiological." This means that it's a normal discharge and doesn't need treating (as is often the case just before and after menstruation).

If the discharge doesn't look normal, see your doctor or gynecologist. Try the following treatment (three pellets of the remedy or remedies you have selected), but be sure to see your doctor if improvement is not rapid.

Depending on the color:
- for discharge that looks like egg white,
  > BORAX 9 C.

- like water,
    SYPHILINUM 9 C.
- greenish discharge,
    MERCURIUS SOLUBILIS 9 C.
- brown or blood-streaked discharge,
  (See your doctor.)
    NITRICUM ACIDUM 9 C.
- yellow or cream-colored discharge,
    PULSATILLA 9 C.
- starchy discharge,
    SABINA 9 C.

Depending on the flow:
- heavy flow,
    ALUMINA 9 C.
- predominantly during the day,
    ALUMINA 9 C.
- predominantly at night,
    MERCURIUS SOLUBILIS 9 C.

Depending on irritation:
- if discharge is yellow and highly
  irritating,
    CREOSOTUM 9 C.
- if it's yellow and non-irritating,
    PULSATILLA 9 C.

For white vaginal discharge in very young women,
    CUBEBA OFFICINALIS 9 C.

If the discharge soils the clothes or smells bad,
    CREOSOTUM 9 C.

Vaginismus

WARNING: Check with your doctor.

A spasmodic contraction of the vagina which makes intercourse impossible or very painful.
Your doctor may prescribe:
    IGNATIA AMARA 9 C,
    PLATINUM METALLICUM 9 C,
    alternate three pellets of each,
    three times a day.

Vaginitis

WARNING: Check with your gynecologist.
An infection of the mucous membranes of the vagina, often caused by bacteria, yeast, or trichomonas.

▷ *See* **Candidiasis, Vaginal discharge.**

When suffering from bartholinitis (inflammation of one of the lubrication glands in the vagina), your doctor may prescribe:
    HEPAR SULPHURIS CALCAREUM 9 C,
    PYROGENIUM 9 C,
    alternate three pellets of each,
    three times a day.

Valeriana officinalis

Base substance: the root of the Valerian plant.

Characteristic symptoms:
Moodiness; muscle spasms; cramp-like pains; fainting due to pain; abdominal bloating of nervous or emotional origin; joint pain, relieved by walking; symptoms aggravated when patient is seated.

Main clinical uses:
Nervous fainting: *WARNING - This disease is serious. Contact your physician immediately for treatment recommendation.*
Nervous joint pains; spasmodic asthma; abdominal bloating.

Varicocele

A varicose (dilated) vein of the spermatic cord, causing a boggy lump in the scrotum. You must absolutely see a doctor.

Varicose veins

Once varicose veins have formed, they cannot be eliminated by homeopathic treatment or probably by any medical treatment for very long. You can only effectively treat the symptoms they cause (swelling, congestion, itching, etc.).

Alternate:
HAMAMELIS VIRGINICA 3 C,
AESCULUS HIPPOCASTANUM 3 C,
three pellets of each, three times a day, twenty days a month during hot weather.

Walking is allowed, but standing in one place for a long time is not recommended. Having varicose veins removed is illogical.

▷ *See* **Sclerosing Injections of varicose veins and hemorrhoids, Suppressing a disease.**

▷ *Also see* **Ulcers.**

Veins

▷ *See* **Phlebitis, Ulcers, Varicose veins.**

Venereal diseases

▷ *See* **Blennorrhagia, Syphilis.**

Veratrum album

Base substance: dried root of White hellebore.

Characteristic signs and symptoms:
Fainting with prostration; tendency to delirium; generalized icy coldness of the skin; cold sweating; vomiting; large amounts of diarrhea; menstrual period pains (cramps).

Main clinical uses:
Diarrhea; menstrual cramps.

Veratrum viride

Base substance: American white hellebore, also known as Wolfbane.

Main clinical uses:
Slow pulse: *WARNING - This disease is serious. Contact your physician immediately for treatment recommendation.*
Cerebral vascular congestion with pain in the occipital region; congested face.

Verbascum thapsus

Base substance: Mullein, also known as Hare's beard.

Main clinical use:
Facial neuralgia with a pinching sensation recurring at a fixed time.

Vertigo

When everything seems to be spinning around you (objective vertigo) or when you have the impression that you're spinning around (subjective vertigo).

WARNING: Check with a doctor if symptoms persist.

Take three pellets of one of the following remedies three times a day.
- vertigo at the slightest movement,
 BRYONIA ALBA 9 C.
- when moving your eyes,
 BRYONIA ALBA 9 C.
- when seeing objects or other people moving,
 COCCULUS INDICUS 9 C.
- when riding in a car,
 COCCULUS INDICUS 9 C.
- on lying down,
 CONIUM MACULATUM 9 C.
- relieved by closing the eyes,
 CONIUM MACULATUM 9 C.
- after eating,
 NUX VOMICA 9 C.

"Fear of heights" is a different ailment and has nothing to do with vertigo. If you must go to the mountains, be on a high balcony or a roof, take:
ARGENTUM NITRICUM 9 C,
three pellets every hour or three times a day depending on circumstances.

Vexation (Consequences of)

▷ *See* **Emotion**.

Viburnum opulus

Base substance: the High bush, also known as High bush cranberry.

Main clinical use:
Painful menstrual periods which last only a few hours.

Vinca minor

Base substance: Wintergreen, also known as Periwinkle.

Characteristic signs and symptoms:
Scalp rash with red skin that is sensitive to the touch; overly oily scalp (hair sticks together); loss of hair in round patches; hair that grows back gray.

Main clinical uses:
Eczema of the scalp; cradle cap.

Viola odorata

Base substance: Sweet Violet.

Main clinical use:
A sensation of broken bones, especially in the wrist.

Viola tricolor

Base substance: Pansy.

Characteristic signs and symptoms:
Purulent rash; enuresis with strong-smelling urine.

Main clinical uses:
Impetigo; enuresis (bed-wetting): *WARNING - These diseases are serious. You should consult your physician for advice.*
Eczema; cradle cap.

Vipera redii

Base substance: Snake venom.

Characteristic signs and symptoms:
Inflammation of superficial veins; swelling of the limbs; pain aggravated when legs are dangling.

Main clinical uses:
Varicose veins; periphlebitis.

Viral hepatitis

WARNING: You must be examined and diagnosed by a doctor. If complications occur, it is easier to handle them when an exact diagnosis of the type of hepatitis is known.

There is no specific treatment for viral hepatitis besides rest and a restricted diet.
Your doctor may prescribe:
CHELIDONIUM MAJUS 9 C,
PHOSPHORUS 7 C,
PHOSPHORUS 9 C,
alternate three pellets of each, three times a day.
Talking to a homeopathic physician will ensure true "individualization" so that the remedies will be chosen with respect to your own particular symptoms of hepatitis.

Viscum album

Base substance: Mistletoe.

Main clinical uses:
Low blood pressure; slow pulse:
*WARNING - These diseases are
serious. You should consult your
physician for advice.*
Dizziness; shortness of breath; fatigue.

Vitiligo (Piebald skin)

Decoloration of the skin, which loses
its pigment in patches. It is harmless
although not always attractive to the
eyes of the patient.
Avoid overexposure to the sun—this
will only make the vitiligo more
apparent. Homeopathy unfortunately
does not offer an effective cure or
treatment for this illness.
It is the experience of the author that
the reputation of AMNI MAJUS 3 X,
(three pellets three times a day for
several months) is overrated.

Vital energy

▷ *See* **Dynamism.**

Vomiting

Take three pellets of the appropriate
remedy every fifteen minutes, every
hour, or three times a day depending
on the intensity of the symptoms.
Check with a doctor if you don't
obtain quick results.
● in case of vomiting and a heavily
coated tongue (tongue is covered with
a thick white film),
     ANTIMONIUM CRUDUM 9 C.
● foul-smelling vomit,
     ARSENICUM ALBUM 9 C.

● patient brings up water immediately
after drinking it,
     ARSENICUM ALBUM 9 C.
● vomiting of mucus, phlegm,
     IPECAC 9 C.
● vomiting and an uncoated tongue,
     IPECAC 9 C.
● vomiting of bile, (See your doctor.)
     IRIS VERSICOLOR 9 C.
● tongue that is coated only toward
the back,
     NUX VOMICA 9 C.
● vomiting of water a short time after
it's been swallowed,
     PHOSPHORUS 9 C.

▷ *Also see* **Nausea.**

Warts

Unless your doctor absolutely advises
it, do not have warts removed. They
may easily grow back (often in greater
number than before), leave visible
scars, or become infected.
The homeopathic treatment acts more
slowly but when the warts have gone,
they should never come back again. If
you have had warts for some time,
you should check with your
homeopathic physician. The treatment
may be long (several months if the
warts have been present for a few
years) but at some point, they will
begin to dry up, darken, and disappear
without leaving a scar. This may take
less than two weeks but it will only
begin once the person's terrain has
been modified.

If the warts made their appearance only recently, you may try three pellets of one or more of the following remedies three times a day.

General treatment

Depending on the physical appearance of the warts:
- if they have a rough, horny appearance,
     ANTIMONIUM CRUDUM 9 C.
- for smooth, flat warts,
     DULCAMARA 9 C.
- for yellow warts, or if the healthy skin surrounding them is yellow,
     NITRICUM ACIDUM 9 C.
- for pedunculated warts (warts on a stalk or stem),
     NITRICUM ACIDUM 9 C.
- for cracked warts,
     NITRICUM ACIDUM 9 C.
- for painful warts,
     NITRICUM ACIDUM 9 C.
- for warts with a cauliflower-like appearance,
     STAPHYSAGRIA 9 C.
- for soft warts,
     THUJA OCCIDENTALIS 9 C.
- for reddish or brownish warts,
     THUJA OCCIDENTALIS 9 C.
- for torn or rough-edged warts,
     THUJA OCCIDENTALIS 9 C.
- for very large warts,
     THUJA OCCIDENTALIS 9 C.

Depending on the location:
Armpit:
     SEPIA 9 C.

Anal region:
     THUJA OCCIDENTALIS 9 C.
▷ *Also see* **Condylomata.**

Back:
     NITRICUM ACIDUM 9 C.

Face, eyelids:
     CAUSTICUM ANNUUM 9 C.

Lips:
     NITRICUM ACIDUM 9 C.

Nose:
     CAUSTICUM ANNUUM 9 C.

Chin:
     THUJA OCCIDENTALIS 9 C.

Hands, back:
     RUTA GRAVEOLENS 9 C.

Palms:
     ANTIMONIUM CRUDUM 9 C.

Nails (around and underneath):
     CAUSTICUM 9 C.

Genitals:
     SABINA 9 C.

Soles of the feet:
     ANTIMONIUM CRUDUM 9 C.

Chest:
     NITRICUM ACIDUM 9 C.

Local treatment

This isn't indispensable but it may be helpful. You may apply THUJA OCCIDENTALIS M.T. twice a day, or the yellow juice of CHELIDONIUM MAJUS (celandine) which is found growing down country lanes or on old stone walls.

If you obtain no results at the end of one month, check with a homeopathic physician. A long-term treatment may be advisable.

Wasps (Stings)

▷ *See* **Insect bites.**

Watering of the eyes

Chronic watering of the eyes may be caused by various factors. Check with your physician or eye doctor.
If this condition started recently, take:
     CONIUM MACULATUM 9 C,
     EUPHRASIA OFFICINALIS 9 C,
     alternate three pellets of each,
     three times a day.

▷ *Also see* **Eyes.**

Weakness

▷ *See* **Fatigue.**

Weaning

▷ *See* **Breast-feeding.**

Wet dreams

▷ *See* **Sexual disorders.**

When to take the Medicine you have been Prescribed

Generally speaking, the following schedule is the most usual one for homeopathic medicines:

• unit-dose tubes should be taken in the morning one hour before breakfast on the date designated by the doctor,

• pellets and/or tablets should be taken thirty minutes before meals (or at least ten minutes before), unless otherwise indicated. When several medicines are indicated, alternate them (take one and then the other) at fifteen-minute intervals.

▷ *See* **Homeopathic medicines, Prescriptions.**

Whitlow (Felon)

A purulent (with pus) infection or abscess at the end of a finger; may involve the fingernail. Occasionally caused by the prick of a thorn or other pointed object.

General treatment:
DIOSCOREA VILLOSA 9 C,
HEPAR SULPHURIS CALCAREUM 9 C,
alternate three pellets of each,
three times a day.

Local treatment:
CALENDULA M.T.,
dissolve twenty-five drops in hot water and bathe your hand.

WARNING: If symptoms persist, discontinue use of the above remedies and consult your physician.

Whooping cough (Pertussis)

Whooping cough may be treatable by Homeopathy, provided the homeopathic physician feels comfortable and experienced enough to do so.

Whooping cough is a respiratory disease, especially of young children. As its name indicates, the disease causes a characteristic "brassy horn" sound when the child breathes in, followed by a cough.

WARNING: If an infant contracts this disease, you should immediately contact your physician or pediatrician.

Willpower

The will to be cured is a basic condition for anyone wishing to heal themselves by Homeopathy. Homeopathy is *demanding;* it can only be applied well if the patient has the necessary capacity of self-observation to find and describe his or her symptoms.

With your cooperation, the homeopathic doctor can help you get well with the right medicines. Homeopathy requires prudence (respecting the laws of Nature, avoiding non-essential procedures) and patience (a persistent ailment cannot usually be cured in a dramatic way).

For lack of willpower, ▷ *see* **Abulia.**

A feeling of possessing two contradictory wills,
ANACARDIUM ORIENTALE 9 C,
three pellets three times a day.

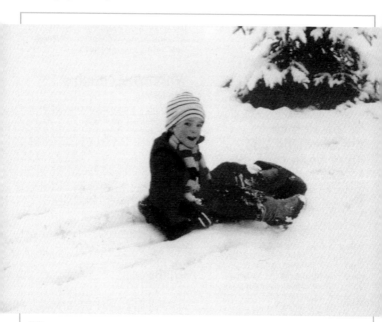

Winter

Wind (Exposure to)

For troubles caused by being out in the wind (colds, runny nose, skin problems, etc.), take three pellets a day of one of the following remedies:
- troubles caused by cold, dry wind,
  ACONITUM NAPELLUS 9 C.
- caused by hot wind,
  ARSENICUM IODATUM 9 C.
- caused by humid wind,
  DULCAMARA 9 C.

Winter

Make sure you're well prepared for the winter.
To prevent the flu and flu-like symptoms, take:
  INLUENZINUM 30 C,
  one weekly unit-dose tube.
Add three pellets of one or more of the following remedies once a week:
  TUBERCULINUM NOSODE 30 C,
  to prevent colds.
  PSORINUM 30 C,
  for particularly cold-sensitive individuals. (Do not use if you have a history of eczema).

Wisdom teeth
(Accidents involving the)

▷ *See* **Teeth.**

Worms (Intestinal)

WARNING: Check with your doctor.
For *symptoms* caused by worms in the intestines, your doctor may prescribe three pellets of one of the following remedies three times a day:
- nervousness caused by worms,
  CINA 9 C.
- itching of the nose,
  CINA 9 C.
- intense hunger,
  CINA 9 C.
- abdominal pains caused by worms,
  SPIGELIA 9 C.
- anal itching,
  TEUCRIUM MARUM VERUM 9 C.

You will also need a chemical medicine treatment to kill the worms, and a homeopathic long-term treatment to prevent their return.

Wrist (Pain in the)

Look under the heading, **Rheumatism,** and supplement the appropriate treatment with:
RUTA GRAVEOLENS 9 C,
three pellets three times a day.

Wryneck (Torticollis, Stiff neck)

Rheumatic (symptomatic) wryneck, due to steady pain and involuntary inaction of neck muscles. Take:
CIMICIFUGA RACEMOSA 9 C,
ARNICA MONTANA 9 C,
BRYONIA ALBA 9 C,
alternate three pellets of each, three times a day.

Spasmodic wryneck (a rotatory spasm or tic due to repeated contractions of the neck muscles, causing the head to tilt to one side):
NATRUM MURIATICUM 9 C.
three pellets three times a day.

Zincum metallicum

Base substance: Zinc.

Suitable for:
Poorly responsive cases (treatment failures); eruptive skin diseases in which the rash is slow to appear, and is later replaced by nervous or emotional disorders.

Characteristic signs and symptoms:
Continual restlessness, particularly of the feet; general sensation of "pins and needles"; convulsions; mental or emotional disorders while suffering from acute disease; intolerance to wine.

Main clinical uses:
Restless legs (constantly moving about, can't remain still); varicose veins; difficulty for eruptive skin diseases to declare themselves.

Appendix:

POTENCY LEVELS

According to the recommendations of the Homeopathic Pharmacopoeia of the United States (H.P.U.S.) for oral dosage forms, the base substances mentioned in *The Guide* should only be used in potencies higher than those listed below: (For example, Aconitum should not be used in a potency under 3 X; one would use 6 X or 12 X - never 1 X or 2 X. Base substances, in some instances, may be toxic.) See **Danger in Homeopathy.**

- Abies canadensis .... 1 X	- Cactus grandiflorus .... 3 X
- Abies nigra .... 1 X	- Calcarea carbonica .... 1 X
- Aconitum napellus .... 3 X	- Calcarea fluorica .... 3 X
- Aesculus hippocastanum .... 1 X	- Calcarea phosphorica .... 1 X
- Aethusa cynapium .... 3 X	- Calendula officinalis .... 1 X
- Agaricus muscarius .... 2 X	- Camphora .... 3 X
- Agraphis nutans .... 1 X	- Cantharis .... 3 X
- Aletris farinosa .... 1 X	- Capsicum annuum .... 3 X
- Allium cepa .... 1 X	- Carbo vegetabilis .... 1 X
- Aloe socotrina .... 1 X	- Carduus marianus .... 1 X
- Alumina .... 3 X	- Caulophyllum thalictroides .... 3 X
- Anacardium orientale .... 3 X	- Causticum .... 2 X
- Anthracinum .... 2 X	- Ceanothus americanus .... 1 X
- Antimonium crudum .... 3 X	- Cedron .... 1 X
- Antimonium tartaricum .... 3 X	- Chamomilla .... 1 X
- Apis mellifica .... 1 X	- Cheiranthus cheiri .... 3 X
- Argentum nitricum .... 6 X	- Chelidonium majus .... 1 X
- Arnica montana (by mouth) .... 3 X	- Chimaphila umbellata .... 1 X
- Arnica montana (externally) ...... 1 X	- Chionanthus virginicus .... 1 X
- Arsenicum album .... 6 X	- Cicuta virosa .... 3 X
- Artemisia abrotanum .... 1 X	- Cimicifuga racemosa .... 1 X
- Arum triphyllum .... 1 X	- Cina .... 1 X
- Asafoetida .... 1 X	- Cinchona officinalis .... 3 X
- Aurum metallicum .... 3 X	- Cistus canadensis .... 1 X
	- Cocculus indicus .... 3 X
- Baryta carbonica .... 6 X	- Coccus cacti .... 2 X
- Belladonna .... 3 X	- Coffea cruda .... 1 X
- Benzoicum acidum .... 2 X	- Colchicum autumnale .... 3 X
- Berberis vulgaris .... 1 X	- Collinsonia canadensis .... 1 X
- Bromium .... 6 X	- Colocynthis .... 3 X
- Bryonia alba .... 3 X	- Conium maculatum .... 3 X

We would like to express our thanks to AIR FRANCE for giving us permission to use their documents (p. 228).

Photos
Agency Createc p. 57, 99, 178, 222, 244.
Agency Explorer p. 18, 39, 51, 57, 62, 72, 77, 82, 115, 130, 132, 145, 174, 182, 185, 188, 194, 200, 233.
Agency Fotogram p. 19, 168.
Agency Vloo p. 29.
Agency La Photothèque p. 67.
Agency Petit Format p. 210.

HEALTH and HOMEOPATHY Publishing, Inc.
P.O. Box 6004
ARLINGTON Va 22206

Achevé d'imprimer par l'Imprimerie Darantiere – 21800 Dijon-Quetigny
ISBN 0-9616 800-0-8 – Dépôt légal n° 35594 – may 2005 – Printed in France